SEEDS OF CHANGE

WOMEN CULTIVATING FOOD SOVEREIGNTY IN HAWAI'I AND AOTEAROA

MONIQUE MIRONESCO

COMMON GROUND

First published in 2025
as part of the **Food Studies Research Network**

Common Ground Research Networks
University of Illinois Research Park
2001 South First Dr, Suite 201 L
Champaign, IL 61820 USA

Library of Congress Cataloging-in-Publication Data

Names: Mironesco, Monique author
Title: Seeds of change : women cultivating food sovereignty in Hawai'i and Aotearoa / Monique Mironesco, Ph.D.
Description: Champaign, IL : Common Ground Research Networks, 2025. | Includes bibliographical references. | Summary: ""Seeds of Change" is organized thematically, weaving together the Hawai'i and Aotearoa New Zealand research to compare and contrast similarities and differences in women's roles and leadership in alternative food networks. More specifically, how does women's leadership in these sites of resistance to the industrial agro-food system work in opposition to the settler colonial context? How do Indigenous and marginalized women's roles play a part in shaping that resistance? How do Indigenous understandings of ecosystems influence the forms of resistance as seen through agricultural and food system practices, both ancient and modern? There is a rich literature on alternative food networks. In recent years however, critiques of alternative food networks as elitist have also come to light. How do Indigenous women resist against those oppressions as well as those coming from the industrial agro-food system? These questions are likely to have different answers in different geographical, political, social and economic contexts, but can nonetheless provide useful models for best practices in other island contexts and beyond. The book focuses on three key themes: 1. Women's leadership in alternative food networks, 2. Centers Indigenous and potentially marginalized voices and stories, 3. Provides a solution-oriented to provide best practices resources from island ecosystems in Hawai'i and Aotearoa to share among AFNs everywhere, but specifically throughout Oceania. I started the research work in Hawai'i in 2019 and went to Aotearoa New Zealand in early 2020, just prior to the Covid-19 pandemic, choosing these two colonized places for the research to reflect American and British imperialist ambitions respectively. I interviewed 29 women in Hawai'i and 19 women in Aotearoa New Zealand; among them female farmers, food system professionals, farmers' union leaders, farmers' market organizers and vendors, self-described compost nerds, nutrition experts, and teachers to name a few, to understand their visions of alternative and more environmentally and socially just food systems. Many of these women work for non-profit organizations working in and around food systems in both places, and they all have networks through which to disseminate information about the book. Indeed, some of the interviewees have access to much larger networks of food system actors than I do. I would be happy to share the book with them and ask them to advertise the book since part of the project is to create an actionable toolkit for food system actors. Disseminating the information embedded in the stories is an important outcome of the project"-- Provided by publisher.
Identifiers: LCCN 2025009668 (print) | LCCN 2025009669 (ebook) | ISBN 9781966214502 hardback | ISBN 9781966214519 paperback | ISBN 9781966214526 adobe pdf
Subjects: LCSH: Women in agriculture--Hawaii | Women in agriculture--New Zealand | Sustainable agriculture--Hawaii | Sustainable agriculture--New Zealand | Food supply--Environmental aspects--Hawaii | Food supply--Environmental aspects--New Zealand
Classification: LCC HD6077.2.P16 M57 2025 (print) | LCC HD6077.2.P16 (ebook) | DDC 338.1082--dc23/eng/20250509
LC record available at https://lccn.loc.gov/2025009668
LC ebook record available at https://lccn.loc.gov/2025009669

ISBN: 978-1-966214-50-2 (HBK)
ISBN: 978-1-966214-51-9 (PBK)
ISBN: 978-1-966214-52-6 (PDF)

TABLE OF CONTENTS

ACKNOWLEDGMENTS

Writing a book during the COVID-19 pandemic might seem like a solitary endeavor, but that was not the case for this project. First and foremost, this book would not exist without the stories shared with me by the incredible women I had the privilege of talking story with, both in Hawai'i and in Aotearoa. Some of them I had been working with for decades through experiential learning projects with my University of Hawai'i West O'ahu students, while others generously shared their stories with me, even though we had never met before. The gratitude I feel for being both a repository and amplifier of these stories is beyond measure. Every story shared was a gift—an abundance that is truly magical.

I could not have completed the interviews in Aotearoa without the guidance of Kate Cherrington, whom I consider my fairy godmother of research. While she was a participant in the study herself, she also introduced me to other women willing to share their experiences. Her support extended beyond research—she checked in on me every few days while I was on the road, made sure I was all right, shared in my frustration when my rental camper van kept overheating, and even booked me a night in a Wellington hotel so I could finally take an "everything shower." We also spent an evening sharing oysters, rosé, and plenty of laughter. What a treasure of a human being. I'm also deeply grateful to Gary Maunakea-Forth of MA'O Farms in Wai'anae, a longtime friend, who first connected me with Kate. I couldn't have done this without either of you.

Phillip Kalantzis-Cope, the editor at Common Ground Press, rescued this book from obscurity and has been a kind and patient colleague throughout the process. His idea for the title made the final cut—thank goodness, because my original version was much too wordy before he worked his editorial magic. Anna Sampaio and Aaron Javsicas also provided valuable theoretical and publishing guidance. Even though we didn't end up working together on the final publication, I truly appreciate the time and attention they gave to shaping this book. The anonymous peer reviewers offered much-needed feedback that sharpened my arguments. Any errors or misinterpretations of their insights are, of course, my own.

Sarah O'Brien was an exceptional developmental editor, refining the language, improving readability, and providing detailed feedback on two drafts of the manuscript. Part of her work was supported by my UHWO colleague Albie Miles's Kellogg Foundation grant focused on sustainable food systems knowledge products—this book certainly fits that vision. Monica LaBriola was an invaluable sounding board, helping me navigate conceptual challenges, especially when we walked the trails together. I hope I was able to support your book project as much as you supported mine.

My mom, Sandra, consistently asked how the book was coming along. While I may have seemed annoyed at times, I truly appreciated her thoughtful attention—it motivated me to finish more than she knows. My daughter, Megan, who was finishing college at the time and then traveling the world making wine, also checked in on the book—when she remembered to text me back. My son, Wyatt, and I turned the process into a friendly competition, comparing daily word counts—me for the book, him for his college papers. I think I got him in the end. And to Mike, who kept the house from disintegrating while I focused on writing. Strangely enough, getting divorced might be the best thing we've done for each other—besides having our kids. Best ex-husband and friend ever.

The "Girl Gang & Trophy Husbands" surf report group chat was steadfast in their encouragement, cheering me on throughout both the writing and publication process. They hyped up my page count, even when I was drowning in imposter syndrome.

Finally, to eighteen years' worth of *Politics of Food* and *Politics of Water* students at UH West Oʻahu—your enthusiasm for these courses fuels me every semester. Your energy and curiosity make me want to be part of the food system transformation project toward a more sustainable, community-focused, local, and just food system.

NOTES ON LANGUAGE

It is time for each one of us to make the commitment to transcend colonialism as people, and for us to work together as peoples to become forces of Indigenous truth against the lie of colonialism. We do not need to wait for the colonizer to provide us with money or to validate our vision of a free future; we only need to start to use our Indigenous languages to frame our thoughts, the ethical framework of our philosophies to make decisions and to use our laws and institutions to govern ourselves.
(Gerald Taiaiake Alfred and Jeff Corntassel 2005)

Food systems provide a space to interrogate white privilege and examine allyship processes within movements working for environmental justice in underserved communities. As a non-Indigenous researcher in a settler colonial space, I recognize the need to attend carefully to distinctions of terminology. In order to ensure equal treatment of different types of writing and languages, this book includes a glossary that brings together key words not only of 'Ōlelo Hawai'i (Hawaiian language) and Te Reo Māori (Māori language) terms, but also of basic "alternative food network," intersectionality, and feminist political ecology theoretical terms—to show that these are indeed different vocabularies—all worthy of equal consideration. Because language has the power to name, challenge, resist, and oppress, we must carefully attend to its many meanings. The readers are invited to learn these special (not necessarily foreign) languages. Including a glossary placing all of these terms on an equal footing indicates the equivalent value placed on these different languages and reinforces the importance of knowledge production coming from all sorts of people, places, and perspectives by revealing the ways in which terms from one language can fill in the gaps left by another. Similarly, the narratives discussed in this book are valuable sources of knowledge and information. In a conscious departure from Chicago Manual of Style (CMS) author-date format, I have included a list of interviewees, with their job titles at the time of the interviews. I have included them as references in the text as well, formatted the same way as academic sources. Their stories and knowledge are equally important and should be recognized as such.

Kanaka Maoli (Native Hawaiian) scholars have called for *not* italicizing *'Ōlelo Hawai'i* (Hawaiian language) words as a way to honor the voices of their ancestors and traditions. Noenoe Silva argues that this typographical choice "resist[s] making the native tongue appear foreign in writing produced in and about a native land and people" (Silva 2004, 13) and normalizes 'Ōlelo Hawai'i as a part of academic discourse. I value and appreciate this call to action, yet as a non-Indigenous scholar in a settler colonial state, following this convention seems misleading on my part and risks cultural appropriation because the language is not my own. It is not my place to insist on conventions about which I should have no input and I cannot speak for others who can very eloquently speak for themselves. However, I see italics as honoring and highlighting the importance of understanding Native words and phrases for non-Native readers. To this end, I have decided on a compromise: Hawaiian or Māori words or phrases are italicized on their first mention in the text and are subsequently not italicized in the rest of the book.

Indigenous scholars have done and continue to do work to address injustices through language reclamation in processes that are nothing short of miraculous. Haunani-Kay Trask, Lilikalā Kameʻeleihiwa, Noenoe Silva, Noelani Goodyear-Kāʻopua, and others in Hawaiʻi, and Linda Tuhiwai Smith, Patricia Johnston, and Leonie Pihama in Aotearoa New Zealand, among many other scholars throughout Oceania, have all contributed to reclaiming history and stories from Indigenous perspectives, using original language sources to highlight resistance to colonial oppression in the past and present. The resistance of the future will stand on this work.

Following Fellezs (2019), I use the term *Kanaka Maoli* to identify Native Hawaiian people. Kanaka Maoli means "the true people" and I use the term interchangeably with Native Hawaiian. I do not use other common terms for Native Hawaiian people, such as *Kanaka ʻŌiwi* (People of the bone), because none of the interviewees used that terminology. I capitalize the word Native in Native Hawaiian to identify and highlight Kanaka Maoli people. In addition, I use Noelani J. Goodyear-Kaʻōpua's convention for Kanaka Maoli "when writing in the singular and undifferentiated plural. *Kānaka Maoli*, with the macron above the *a*, is used when the number of Native Hawaiians is…a known quantity" (Fellezs 2019). With respect to Aotearoa New Zealand, per Bartos, it is "common for academic literature to cite both the Indigenous and settler term for the country: Aotearoa New Zealand. The combination of the two terms draws attention to the contentiousness of colonial histories and the resulting multiple ethnicities and identities prevalent throughout the country today" (2016, 92). I follow these conventions to account for the ongoing processes of settler colonialism in this particular geographic region and political framework.

Alfred and Corntassel famously insisted in 2005 that Indigenous studies scholars understand terms like "Native sovereignty" as "Western conceptions, with their own philosophical distance from the natural world, [that] have more often reflected kinds of structures of coercion and social power…Indigenous philosophies are premised on the belief that the human relationship to the earth is primarily one of partnership" (45). Jarosz (2014) aptly interprets this to mean that the term "food sovereignty" is equally fraught and not necessarily a useful or even accurate way of describing people's relationship to land or food because "[w]hite Euro-American understandings of sovereignty commonly encompass concepts such as nation, state, boundary, territory, and citizen" (231). This conception shifts the focus—and, more importantly the responsibility—to the individual and to Indigenous communities to claim their rights to self-determination without providing any tools for moving in that direction or crafting any kind of a plan for concrete action. To be sure, self-determination is critical to Indigenous rights, be they related to food, land, or other issues, but the language of the "individual" and the "self" is not as culturally appropriate in this context, given its fraught political and historical (read: colonial) antecedents. Focusing instead on communal and collaborative aspects of life can shift the narrative away from personal choice and consumption within an insatiable capitalist system. Coté (2016) suggests that "indigenizing" the food sovereignty debate can move us toward "emphasizing cultural responsibilities and relationships that indigenous peoples have with their environment" (13), which would enable Indigenous peoples to assert control over their own communities' health and well-being through the decolonization process. She cites Indigenous scholar Waziyatawin's assertion that

> [t]he more we learn to restore local food practices, the more likely we are to defend those practices and the stronger our cultural ties to our homeland become. If we choose this course of action, we can simultaneously engage in both the resurgence and resistance elements of a decolonization movement. (15)

Similarly, LaDuke (2005) argues that a "recovery of the people is tied to the recovery of the food" (210). In this sense, then, healthy and culturally relevant food fosters connections to history, genealogy, and land. Until a more useful lexicon emerges that includes Indigenous perspectives of self-determination around food system issues, food sovereignty as the term of choice will have to suffice.

An additional distinction between "food sovereignty" and "food security" should be made here as a preface to the larger discussion of the relationship between food sovereignty and Indigenous values. The language of food sovereignty asserts self-determination as its goal, reducing the emphasis in the discourse of food security on deficits within Indigenous communities (Wiebe and Wipf 2011), instead emphasizing control and leadership over narratives of abundance and redefining cultural practices to include attention to wealth of both spirit and health (Shattuck et al. 2015). Food sovereignty focuses on an assets-based (rather than a deficit-based) model of the food system, and renounces discussions of food security in response to food deserts by asserting the independence and self-determination of Indigenous and marginalized communities to engage in long-standing sustainable agricultural practices based on tending and nourishing soils and peoples. That said, talking about the ingenuity of Indigenous food and agricultural systems runs the risk of cultural appropriation if it is not placed within the larger context of a Land Back movement—a push by Indigenous peoples around the world for restitution of stolen lands to ensure a path toward self-determination, environmental sustainability, and economic well-being (David Suzuki Foundation 2023). For example, Kate Cherrington, one of my interviewees in Aotearoa New Zealand and the chair of the Te Pūtea Whakatupu Trust (now known as Tapuwae Roa), explains: "when I look at those systems, the non-Indigenous food systems and of course they're all falling apart. And then they'll come to us and say, can you help us today? Help us figure this out?" (Cherrington 2020). Policies that ignore or sidestep Indigenous land dispossession through colonization and the resulting demands of the Land Back movement are likely to be met with resistance or even derision, especially as they relate to the food system. As Rudolph and McLachlan demonstrate in the Canadian context (2013), importing shelf-stable foods into Indigenous communities has led to many diet-related illnesses. In many settler colonial contexts, historical injustices and the privileging of resource extraction, military funding, construction, or tourism at the expense of traditional foodways have shaped resistance in the form *relational* alternative food systems focused on environmental justice, and food sovereignty through community and capacity-building. Lemke and Delormier (2017) argue that a combination of western and Indigenous practices geared toward food system balance can "provide tools for social movements and communities to challenge existing structural inequalities and leverage social change" (1). Additionally, an agroecological focus on biodiversity mimics Indigenous food systems by focusing on community and sustainability (Stein et al. 2018). Understanding food system connections has the potential to challenge structural barriers such as land access and fair labor practices, and to provide a space for Indigenous peoples to regenerate their knowledge practices and system (Lemke and Delormier 2017). This well-being is rooted in a deep understanding of ecosystem resources and services through generations of careful observation and scientific inquiry, which in turn produces invaluable traditional ecological knowledge through community-based control of natural resources (Morrison 2011). Kamuela Enos's focus on the restoration of "ancestral abundance" is attentive to Indigenous peoples' relationship to land and their stewardship of it for future generations (2013). What is good for Indigenous peoples, whether Kanaka Maoli or Māori, is good for everyone, and moves society at large toward ecological sustainability.

Developing a critical understanding of how colonialism has shaped life and land in Hawaiʻi and Aotearoa New Zealand can help Kanaka Maoli and Māori communities re-engage with traditions. *Marae* (meeting grounds—places for communal gatherings honoring Māori traditions and practices) in Aotearoa New Zealand provide space to engage in this process with support and care due to their *ahikāroa* (connection to place), *whakapapa* (genealogy), and connection to the *whenua* (land and environment) (Moorfield 2024). As Moeke-Pickering et al. (2015) have argued, many of the solutions that would engender Māori food sovereignty and access can be sourced from Māori communities and knowledge bases through the application of Māori worldviews and principles. To add another analytical layer to these points, some women in certain *iwi* (tribe)*, hapū* (sub tribe), or even *whānau* (extended family or kinship group) have more power than in others (Cherrington 2020; Mules 2020), and many of the struggles that Māori women face or have been engaged in are based on re-centering a Māori worldview of connectedness that appreciates relationships between people, land, diverse species, and spiritual connections to certain places and sustainable ways of living and feeding family and community.

In addition, like most Indigenous groups around the world, Māori do not fit within a single, easy-to-categorize label. In fact, Linda Tuhiwai Smith explains that the

> term Māori only became meaningful as a category because of colonisation. It is the label which was used by colonisers to define the native inhabitants they encountered. It was not the term by which these members of whānau, hapū, and iwi necessarily described themselves. It is as much a political construction as a construction of race. (2019, 41)

Thus, while it is certainly not my place to problematize these terms, it is worth mentioning that Māori feminists and scholars have been doing so for several decades and that while the term Māori is often used throughout this book, it is not without its own attendant colonizer baggage.

This book's central project is to amplify the voices of women leaders who are working to transform food systems in two distinct colonized spaces in Oceania, settled by two different colonizers, the United States and Britain, respectively. They offer two distinct responses to food system change by focusing on the assets within their respective communities—namely on the resilience and strength of the work coming out of these various projects. The original idea for the research came about from two decades of teaching at the University of Hawai'i West O'ahu and doing service-learning in politics of food classes with my students alongside a variety of community partners in our service area of the Leeward Coast and Central O'ahu as well as the North Shore. Speaking with, as it turns out, mostly women, leaders of these organizations, I found that their work was occurring in discrete silos, though that has definitely changed in recent years due to the advent of social media and targeted efforts by some of them to connect with others doing similar work. The focus was not necessarily on decolonizing food systems as a whole, but rather on making a difference in their respective communities. I chose to conduct research in Aotearoa, originally almost as a "foil" to the Hawai'i-based research. By collecting and sharing information and resources, this project brings together voices and finds threads of connectivity to enhance the value of these experiences and stories for all involved. Native scholars have done and continue to do incredible work around many of these issues (Byrd 2011; Deer 2015; Goodyear-Ka'ōpua et al. 2014; LaDuke 1999; Moreton-Robinson 2015; Simpson 2017; Tengan 2008; Trask 1993; Yamashiro and Ka'ōpua 2014). My intention is to bring their work into conversation with some of the pragmatic solutions offered by the respondents in this study. How can this project amplify their voices through the lens of intersectional and anticolonial feminist political ecology and resistance to appropriation?

Defining the limitations of the word "women" is appropriate in this "Notes on Language," given that it is one of the main organizing principles of the book. This label has been destabilized by theorists from various disciplines, starting most famously with Judith Butler (1990). Gendered terms like "women" have given way to "gender non-conforming" or "gender fluid" identities throughout contemporary society. These new terms raise issues when using them as analytical categories in intersectional analysis and praxis. If we cannot rely on stable identity categories, are we bound to lose the opportunity to understand how multiple identity categories interact to form specific types of oppressions, or conversely, to serve as avenues for liberation? Indeed, Sundberg (2017) asks: "if women are no longer the organizing purpose of feminism and gender no longer its central analytical category, then what is the point of FPE [feminist political ecology]" (13)? To simplify, I would call this the "as women" problem. It would be essentialist to use "women" as a singular analytic category, just as it would be essentialist to assign specific perspectives to Indigenous peoples. Clearly, this is not the goal. We cannot assume that there are shared concerns by all women simply due to their gender identity, nor can we assume that there is a single Indigenous viewpoint of food sovereignty or self-determination; perhaps there is an *affinity*, rather than an identity? Attending to this affinity helps us understand how intersectionality can maintain its use of gender as an analytic category, and it means that gender fluidity does not spell the end of intersectional analysis. Gender fluidity does not make intersectional analysis impossible; it just makes it more nuanced and more complex because identity boundaries are constantly moving and shifting, making any analysis necessarily temporary. The interviewees in this project all identified as women because they responded to a call to talk story for "women leaders in alternative food networks." I, thus, follow their lead and identify them as "women" in the book. This does not mean that gender was the only identity category that mattered to them, nor does it mean that their gender identity is not fluid. At the point in time we spoke, they all identified as women, and I respect their decision to do so by privileging their experiences.

   Like "women," the word "colonial" also needs examination and explanation. Nancy Shoemaker (2015) clearly outlines the many variations of colonialism: planter colonialism, extractive colonialism, trade colonialism, transport colonialism, imperial power colonialism, not-in-my-backyard colonialism, legal colonialism, rogue colonialism, missionary colonialism, romantic colonialism, postcolonial colonialism and, of course, settler colonialism. This typology broadly defines the different colonialisms in the context of the turn in the academic literature toward what is now commonly called settler colonialism, which itself also carries different connotations. Lorenzo Veracini, a leading scholar in settler colonial theory, claims that colonialism and settler colonialism are antithetical to each other (2010). Many of these types of colonialism co-exist or even morph into each other in various geographic contexts, especially throughout Oceania. That said, some of these definitions are time-specific and only identify processes that occurred during the nineteenth and early parts of the twentieth century. Nevertheless, in 1999, Kathy Ferguson and Phyllis Turnbull's book *Oh, Say, Can You See? The Semiotics of the Military in Hawai'i* looked toward a twenty-first-century version of colonialism by outlining the ways in which the military is hidden in plain sight in Hawai'i "through the uneasy combination of fears and longings in the colonial encounter" (5). Although they focus specifically on the ongoing militarization and occupation of Hawai'i, the colonial processes in other spaces remain.

When people who live on the continent talk about colonialism, they tend to think of it in the past tense and assume that the US no longer actively colonizes territories. Living in what some might call a "postcolonial" state like Hawai'i, or what others might call occupied land, we witness daily that colonialism is still going strong. From the heavy-duty military vehicles clogging up and damaging the roads, to the freeway exits unproblematically renaming Hawaiian geographic locations to military base names, colonialism is still alive and well in Hawai'i. Perhaps a more useful term, then, is "neocolonialism," which implies that the capitalist system is the means by which imperial powers dominate their colonial subjects. I argue here that Hawai'i and Aotearoa New Zealand are in limbo between colonialism and neocolonialism. The US and Britain still occupy land and territory in both spaces, at the same time as the indirect control implied by neocolonialism continues. As such, I use the terms interchangeably throughout the book, sometimes leaning more on the land and territorial occupation definition inherent in the word colonialism, and other times focusing more on the economic and capitalist aspects of neocolonial processes. Other times, I rely on settler colonial terminology to denote the erasure of Indigenous people in the contexts I describe.

Finally, a note on stylistic choices is warranted here as well. I capitalize the word "Indigenous" throughout the entire book, unless it appears in lowercase in a direct quotation per Younging's 2018 urging in *The Elements of Indigenous Style* as a "deliberate decision that redresses mainstream society's history of regarding Indigenous peoples as having no legitimate national identities; governmental, social, spiritual, or religious institutions; or collective rights" (77). Clearly, the premise of this book supports this stylistic choice as an important one. Moreover, I am choosing to avoid capitalizing the words "western" and "white" when it comes to values and identities, though I am capitalizing other ethnic identifiers.

INTRODUCTION

Food for us comes from our relatives, whether they have wings or fins or roots.
That is how we consider food. Food has a culture. It has a history. It has a story.
It has relationships.
—Winona LaDuke (2012)

This is a story of stories about food. It focuses on women's leadership in alternative food networks (AFNs) in two areas of Oceania: Hawai'i and Aotearoa New Zealand. AFNs are systems of producing and distributing local, organic, and fair-trade foods through alternative means, such as farmers' markets, community-supported agriculture (CSA) schemes, direct-to-consumer sales, farm stands, and u-pick operations (Goodman and Goodman 2009). In contrast, the industrial agro-food system is defined by all the activities and institutions involved in growing, processing, distributing, and consuming food on a large scale, generally via a centralized system. It's a complex network that includes farming, transportation, supermarkets, and even regulatory bodies. This system is usually dominated and controlled by large corporations, which have significant influence over how food is produced and sold. These corporations often prioritize efficiency, profit, and large-scale production (Natural Resources Defense Council 2020). AFNs interrupt power relations to work against the capitalist system's concept of economies of scale as a desirable achievement to increase profits. Instead they work in opposition to the violence against and destruction of ecosystems, polluting practices of industrial agriculture, and firmly against genetic engineering, exploitative labor practices, and large-scale automation of agriculture and other food system components. Although all kinds of people work within and use AFNs, they appeal to women in particular because they provide a deliberative space of engagement and a form of resistance to the industrial agro-food system. They do so by addressing specific situated concerns— intersectional lived experiences—and as such can provide meaningful input for transformative food system projects and policies to support those changes.

   The everyday practices of gender roles impact the processes of establishing and maintaining AFNs. Women play a critical role in creating alternative flows of power and material in everyday life, and their resistance motivates community-based action. AFNs create counterflows of food, knowledge, nourishment, and community and can create intersectional spaces—that is, spaces where experiences, stories, identities, knowledge, and relationships foster potential food system transformation in order to build wealth that is not necessarily based on money or profits, but on a generational wealth of knowledge and understanding of the food system. As island ecosystems in the context of climate change, Hawaiʻi and Aotearoa New Zealand provide key spaces to research how women belonging to different communities, including but not limited to Indigenous and marginalized communities (which are often one and the same), contribute to these processes of resistance and disrupt the settler colonial project by creating alternative visions in the struggles around land, sovereignty, and self-determination.

This book is based on interviews with woman-identifying farmers, food system professionals, public health advocates, nutritionists, food bank and farmer cooperative managers, community organizers working on agricultural and food-justice issues, educators, farmers' union leaders, food waste diversion experts, self-described "compost nerds," as well as farmers' market organizers and vendors. By weaving together and reflecting on these women's narratives, this book considers how AFNs are shaped by women's political, economic, and social experiences as they are altered by gender, race, ethnicity, indigeneity, and class. Using an intersectional feminist political ecology (FPE) framework, it considers how these elements of identity are co-constituted by ecological systems. Intersectionality can be understood as a process or an analytical tool (Collins and Bilge 2020) that focuses on understanding interlocking systems of oppression like politico-legal institutional frameworks, as Patricia Hill Collins explains in her seminal work (1990) on intersectionality. Moreover, Kimberlé Crenshaw (1991) asserts that treating identities as a sum of discrete parts cannot, by definition, either reflect the wholeness of a person, nor can it lead to justice when encountering or interacting with institutional systems. Much of the authoritative literature on intersectionality—from its inception with Crenshaw and Hill Collins's work, to more recent treatments of the topic—still tends to focus on race, class, gender, sexuality, and ethnicity not just as intersecting social identity categories, but with more of a focus on structural inequality and systemic oppression. Crenshaw explained in a *Vox* interview that the "point of intersectionality is to make room for 'more advocacy and remedial practices' to create a more egalitarian system" (Coaston 2019). For example, in a more recent definition of intersectionality, Cho et al. (2013) explain that it consists of three different moves: investigating intersectional dynamics, understanding intersectionality in terms of theory and methodology, and using an intersectional lens for political projects through praxis. While they are not mutually exclusive, this book mostly employs the third perspective. As Cho et al. suggest, intersectionality should be used for what it does, rather than what it is. I expand this definition of intersectionality to include human interaction with nature through food systems and the inclusion of ecosystems as non-human actors as well as Indigenous knowledge systems as told through stories and practiced through actions. This book highlights the voices of Indigenous and marginalized women and their allies through interviews that emphasize Indigenous cosmology, which values knowledge and being as connected. There is a focus on inequality as a through line of intersectionality, rather than only focusing on overlapping social identities to understand multiple modes of subordination that are more than just the sum of their parts. Using qualitative research analysis, I draw out emergent themes within the stories told to me by woman-identifying food system actors in Oceania, examining their perspectives on food system inequality and how those views push them to seek out AFNs to serve not only their shifting and relational identities, but also foster food system transformation.

Some of the narratives in the interviews conducted for this book include essentializing claims about women's "inherent" capacity for food system work. These claims risk adding to women's already overburdened roles—a risk that disproportionately affects women of color or women with fewer material resources. How can an intersectional FPE analysis intervene to answer Juanita Sundberg's (2017) call for "supporting broader feminist political objectives for more equitable and ecologically viable futures" (18)? The book demonstrates these women's potential to shape new models of agricultural communities and provides examples for other geographic and settler colonial contexts. The goal is to create a space through combined stories to build a framework for food system transformation.

In gathering stories of alternative and more environmentally and socially just food systems, this book focuses on the following questions: How does women's leadership in these sites of resistance work in opposition to the settler colonial context? How do Indigenous and marginalized women and their allies shape that resistance? How do Indigenous understandings of ecosystems and Indigenous agricultural and food system practices, both ancient and modern, influence these forms of resistance? A rich literature on AFNs exists, but little of it addresses women's roles from intersectional perspectives. In fact, much of it comes from a deficit perspective, which replicates colonial understandings of Indigenous communities. It invokes the language of resilience, strength, and the capacity to recover from adversity. Access to food should not be considered a concept rooted in adversity; it is a basic need for survival. Nor is it a concept; it is the tangible intake of material substance into the human body, at the very least, and in the best-case scenario, it should also be good, clean, fair, and pleasurable. Rather than focusing on deficits, we should be asking the following questions: What are a community's capacities? What are its assets? What are the available tools to improve food systems? We should focus on what we have, and how we can make the best use of those assets to serve our communities.

Understanding what works in AFNs can help us find ways to scale up projects to benefit greater numbers of communities. In recent decades, critiques of AFNs as elitist have emerged (Guthman 2008; Allen 2004), highlighting that AFNs tend to reach people who already have the means to avail themselves of their resources. CSAs, farmers' markets, farm stands, and even chain health food stores tend to be more expensive than grocery stores or large retailers like Walmart and Costco. How do we retool AFNs to serve both economically and structurally disadvantaged marginalized communities? How do we reshape some of the food system structures that might already be in place to reflect community needs? The women interviewed for this book describe experiences that are not the same, but they are shared. They tell stories of struggle, but also stories of beauty and joy in thriving communities. As an ally, it is my responsibility to amplify the voices of women, from formerly unknown workers to well-known leaders in the food system, in these settler colonial spaces as reflections of resistance within the food system.

To change the relatively limited narrative of food justice, we must not only change the questions we are asking but contextualize them differently. How does intersectional FPE change our understanding of feminist food justice? How do Indigenous women resist various socioeconomic and sociocultural oppressions and those of the industrial agro-food system? These questions have different answers in different geographic, political, social, and economic contexts, but can nonetheless provide useful models for best practices in other island contexts. This book helps to fill a substantial gap in the agro-food literature and feminist scholarship on areas of structural issues and social change by (1) using Oceania as an example of a settler colonial system that disrupted a working independent Indigenous food system (among the many other things it disrupted); and (2) by examining how women leaders there have responded to that disruption by contributing to their own burgeoning alternative food movements.

Existing Scholarship on Alternative Food Networks

The classic literature on AFNs examines how AFNs resist the industrial agro-food system by encouraging the ethical production and consumption of locally grown, organic, and fair-trade foods (Allen 2004; Goodman and Goodman 2009; Hinrichs 2003).

Venn et al. (2006) identify multiple frameworks for AFNs, but the diversity of AFNs has grown even larger since the publication of their article. AFNs are not without their critics. By definition, their agricultural and value-added products tend to be more expensive due to the higher costs of production (it stands to reason that products made or grown with fairly compensated labor will cost more than those produced with exploited labor) and thus are only available to people who are able to pay higher prices. Critics of AFNs tend to focus on how they exclude people of color, Indigenous peoples, and other marginalized communities (Hinrichs 2003; DeLind 2010; Hinrichs and Kremer 2002; Slocum 2007; Guthman 2011; Allen 2004; Edwards-Jones 2010; Rudolph and McLachlan 2013). Research on AFNs that engages with marginalized communities focuses on the supply side, such as getting more healthy food into underserved communities, rather than the racialized injustices that have produced food insecurity in the first place (Alkon and Norgaard 2009). In this same literature, AFNs in the settler colonial context traditionally focus on food deserts rather than community assets, leading some within marginalized communities to resent researchers wanting to exploit their problems (Meyer 2019) for academic gain. The goal is, instead, to focus on giving support to community so they can receive the help *they* want, rather than enduring unwanted "help" that outsiders believe they need.

Some of the literature on AFNs examines women's roles in agricultural households (Whatmore 1991; Lobao and Meyer 1995; Sachs 1996; Meares 1997; Chiappe and Flora 1998; Trauger 2004; Cairns et al. 2010; Castellano 2016). Allen and Sachs (1992) insist on avoiding essentializing women in agriculture and AFNs due to their roles as mothers. However, Spivak's (Danius, Jonsson, and Spivak 1993) strategic essentialism offers a way out of this theoretical impasse by advancing the pragmatic idea of using essentialism as a *temporary* strategy to achieve certain political goals. This move aligns with the intersectional praxis approach to use gender as one of many social categories and is effective in moving the political project of food system transformation forward. The literature on women in AFNs also focuses on their role as consumers. Women tend to be more likely to shop at farmers' markets, to subscribe to CSAs, and to engage in reflexive consumption (DeLind and Ferguson 1999; Little et al. 2009; Cairns et al. 2010). Chiappe and Flora (1998) demonstrate that women's involvement in sustainable agriculture tends to create communities of practice that increase a sense of place and foster relationships through a commitment to social change based around food and agriculture. However, these practices tend to be available to women with privilege because they require significant material resources. Women who work long hours at low-waged jobs may not have time to shop at farmers' markets at set times, buy unprocessed whole foods, or prepare meals from scratch for their families. Although they may be inclined to do so, there are only so many hours in the day, and the ease of shopping at the supermarket at any hour or consuming fast food or easily reheated takeaway is a likely reality. In fact, Castellano (2015, 2016) argues that the time required for AFN food provisioning and cooking, let alone growing food, increases the amount of care work women do for their families and can contribute to a triple burden—on top of working outside the home and the mental and physical load of caring for their families. Although encouraging women to grow food at home or in community gardens benefits individuals, their families, and local communities, and is a critical component of the (re)production of AFNs (Castellano 2016), it also places an additional burden on their lives and reduces the amount of time women can spend on other pursuits.

In its focus on women within farm families and women as consumers, the existing research on AFNs posits a direct relationship between farms and consumers. In the last few decades, AFNs have come to involve much more complex networked connections. In addition, much of the AFN literature focuses either on production (Goodman and DuPuis 2002) or consumption (DeLind and Ferguson 1999; Little et al. 2009; Cairns et al. 2010), paying little attention to the systemic factors that contribute to continued inequality in AFNs. This book engages women as leaders; rather than essentializing their gender, it rethinks their roles as care providers in and out of the home. It focuses on women's leadership in creating and maintaining AFNs that work in specific communities and with specific characteristics throughout Oceania. Island ecosystems in the region demonstrate how closed systems work and how human relationships with food systems and the natural world shape AFNs.

Since Michael Pollan's *Omnivore's Dilemma* hit the mainstream in 2006, terms like "organic," "local," "ethical," and "fair trade," are routinely used by people making food choices based on health concerns and interest in environmental justice, increasing attention to AFNs. Indeed, "consumers who prioritize local foods tend to be concerned with a broader social and environmental mission, expressing concern for farmers, workers, animal welfare, or rebuilding communities" (Adams and Salois 2010; Bean and Sharp 2011, cited in Castellano 2015, 465–466). Participating in AFNs leads to what Nigh and Cabañas (2015) call reflexive consumption: "direct, face-to-face relationships in local markets [that] allows the recognition on both sides of the realities and necessities each party confronts" (322). In some places, governments have encouraged AFNs through policy and legislation. For example, the Appellation d'Origine Contrôlée (AOC) in France indicates a particular region's "*terroir*," or "taste of place" (330). While this is generally applied to how the natural environment, soil, geography, and climactic conditions affect the flavor of grapes for winemaking, it has expanded its applicability to many other food products, including cheese, and even vegetables (Bosco and Joassart-Marcelli 2018; Barber 2015). This emphasis on regionality and local production and consumption allows AFNs to thrive with state assistance and enables various actors to create community and solidarity within AFNs. Nigh and Cabañas (2015) show that there is increased interest in environmental concerns and sustainable agricultural practices, as well as social and economic justice for farmers on the part of government. In addition, many non-governmental organizations are pushing for food system changes and food sovereignty. La Via Campesina, a global peasants' rights organization fighting for both of these goals, identifies five specific points:

> (1) ensuring peasant access to agricultural inputs like land and seeds; (2) nurturing diversified, locally appropriate agricultural practices; (3) protecting and promoting local markets for the products of peasant agriculture; (4) ensuring all citizens' rights to have healthy, locally produced food; and (5) promoting peasants' right to full participation in setting agricultural policy. (Aguayo and Latta 2015, 400)

While much of La Via Campesina's work occurs in the global South, these food sovereignty goals based on AFNs are key to achieving food system change. Their lessons are valid for the context of Oceania in systemic support for AFNs.

Political Engagement and Food Sovereignty

The literature on AFNs proposes two alternatives for defining food sovereignty. The first is intentionally vague, so as to enable communities to define what food sovereignty means for them (Park et al. 2015). In this framework, food sovereignty, which focuses on the control of the means of production, stands in bold contrast to "food security," which focuses on availability and access. In fact, food sovereignty "puts the dominant agro-industrial model in question and converts food into a broader site of political engagement" (see, e.g., Wittman et al. 2010; cited in Aguayo and Latta 2015, 400). This view of political engagement as going beyond individual consumer choice is an important nexus of food system change. Wiebe and Wipf assert that "food sovereignty, thus, contrasts strongly with food security and its supply-side emphasis, a construction that, in turn, generally ignores how power relations determine favoured production, distribution, and consumption patterns within a dominant food system that promotes high-input, intensive production methods" (Wiebe and Wipf [61] as cited in Rudolph and McLachlan 2013, 1080). Food sovereignty holds further implications for Indigenous people that are relevant to this project.

Another definition of food sovereignty is more detailed. Shattuck et al. (2015) rely on the original 2007 La Via Campesina's Declaration of Nyéléni to assert that food sovereignty is "the right of people to healthy and culturally appropriate food produced through ecologically sound and sustainable methods, and their right to define their own food and agriculture systems" (422). They identify inherent tensions within the food sovereignty movement. For example, it is difficult to reconcile the interests of smallholder farmers with those of landless (often migrant or seasonal) rural workers, or the emphasis on providing fair prices for farmers with the needs of poor urban consumers for affordable (but clean and fair) food. As Agarwal (2014) has noted, family farms, especially in the global South, are ripe spaces for imposing and reproducing patriarchal practices due to long-standing cultural traditions. Finally, discussions about food sovereignty in the global South do not always align with those of urban communities in the United States organizing around racial justice. These debates are ongoing and very real—and they represent issues that need to be addressed within this growing movement (Shattuck et al. 2015).

Despite its limitations, the food sovereignty discourse, especially within Indigenous communities, remains an important site of political resistance to the global industrial agro-food system and its capitalist focus on profits over people and the environment. These neoliberal economic policies are entrenched within a neocolonial context. Colonialism continues to have lasting impacts on Indigenous peoples everywhere, and the industrial agro-food system is itself a colonizing force that has reshaped the control of agricultural production and formation of dependent food system relationships. Indigenous scholars have argued that the notion of the "postcolonial" is inherently false and urge us to instead decolonize our diets (Esquibel and Calvo 2013). The loss of land and the decimation of Indigenous peoples through diseases and health disparities are still very real and ongoing effects of the colonial project. There is nothing over and done with about it. Kari Marie Norgaard (2019) critiques the "sudden" discovery within academia of the Anthropocene as a term that acknowledges humans' deleterious impact on the environment, when "an understanding of this relationship between humans and the natural world is only new to some" (230). Native peoples have known for thousands of years that their role within nature is part of a larger web of connections that work together to co-constitute the natural world. Norgaard also argues that "just as Indigenous people experience the absence of traditional foods as a mechanism of forced assimilation, the reorganization of the natural world violently restricts potential gender identities, expressions, and arrangements" (2019, 194). Yet, it is within this complicated context that women have become leaders within the food sovereignty movement. Resistance to these systemic structures of colonial oppression takes many forms. For example, in Chile, the feminist values found in certain organizations meant to support farmers exist in contrast with the traditional values and gender relations in many Mapuche communities (Aguayo and Latta 2015). In their study on Māori women leading sustainable food systems in Aotearoa New Zealand, Stein et al. (2018) detail numerous instances of women's leadership in community, culture, family, and health and find that women's leadership is inherent in self-determination through food sovereignty.

Leadership of Indigenous Women

The ancestral land tenure system in many, though not all, Indigenous communities involves stewardship rather than ownership of land. Land stewardship in Native communities often refers to the land as an ancestor and provides a framework for an ethic of care. Seeing the land as a family member supports the view of humans living *within* ecosystems rather than extracting resources from the land. It encourages humans to avoid doing harm to our relatives, because we cannot separate the well-being of land from the well-being of its inhabitants as active participants in the ecosystem. Creation stories in many Indigenous cultures highlight the bonds between Indigenous peoples and their ancestors, which can take the form of geographic features, specific places, as well as fauna and flora. Women's varied roles in these systems provide nourishment and abundance to the people living within them. Kinship to ancestral lands fosters a sense of responsibility to care for natural resources for future generations (Stein et al. 2018). It also focuses on passing down knowledge to young people so as to maintain the legacy of leadership among younger women. The Indigenous Women's Network (2009) articulated the need to transfer knowledge to new generations: "We need to be able to pass on and acquire new skills and knowledge to new leaders—particularly young women—through our traditional ways of sharing orally and demonstrating in a safe and nurturing atmosphere" (365). If the oft-cited evidence that educating women in developing nations is key to reducing global poverty is accurate (Ban 2013), then it stands to reason that sharing knowledge and skills regarding caring for natural resources with younger generations of women would have a similarly positive effect on protecting lands and soil to grow food sustainably (McIntyre et al. 2009).

The narrative behind the restoration of ancestral abundance is one of plenty and is embodied in the everyday practices of producing and consuming culturally appropriate foods. For example, specific crops are grown as a resistance to colonialism and the global agro-food system. In Hawai'i, growing and consuming *kalo* (taro) is an act of resistance to the importation of ultra-processed foods from the continent. In Aotearoa New Zealand, *kūmara* (sweet potato) has a long history of cultivation by Māori and acts as a challenge to industrial food. As it does with *criollo maize* (native corn) in Mexico, this work

> presents an indirect but powerful challenge to the state's assumption that integration into a global agricultural economy is inherently desirable…the campesinos of the Amecameca Valley continue to articulate an alternative geopolitical logic; pursuing food security by sowing their fields, feeding their families, and nourishing their local markets with criollo maize. (Mulaney 2014, 424)

Women often carry out the work of growing and finding alternative ways to sell maize and kalo, and they express pride in the Indigenous values and stories behind the crops. Whereas kalo might embody resistance in Hawaiian culture, it is fair to say that *'āina* is the organizing core social unit. It is inextricably linked to origin stories and an inherent part of any Native Hawaiian genealogy. 'Āina is often loosely translated as "land" in English, but its true meaning is "that which feeds." While this is not a *kaona*, or hidden meaning of the word, this distinction is significant to understanding the larger interwoven meaning of the word and concept in Native Hawaiian culture, agriculture, sustainability, and the relationality of land, nature, food, and people. One Hawaiian proverb states: *He ali'i ka 'āina,* [the land is chief,] *he kauwā ke kanaka,* [man is its servant]. This *'ōlelo no'eau* (proverb or poetical saying) is a reminder of the *kuleana* (responsibility, privilege, small parcel of land) we have as people to serve 'āina, as well as the reassurance that in return 'āina will care for, feed, and provide for our needs (kaainamomona. org 2025). Unlike the word *"terroir,"* " *'āina* is not a culinary term, but one that reflects Indigenous Hawaiian culture and the land as sustenance" (Costa and Besio 2011, 845, emphasis in original). The meaning of the word "land" in Māori resides in a similar connected relationship between humans and land. Indeed, "the Māori word for land, whenua, also means placenta. All life is seen as being born from the womb of Papatūānuku, under the sea…and tangata whenua—literally, people of the land—are those who have authority in a particular place" (Te Ahukaramū 2007b).

In this framework, women's leadership is crucial in sustainable agriculture practices because it fosters equitable distribution of resources as well as information. People who can do, must do—this is a tenet of people who have been oppressed and who have found hope in educating future generations on the "good life" and passing on knowledge that would otherwise have been lost. That sense of duty may unfairly add yet another responsibility to the many obligations of those who are already oppressed in a variety of ways, but kuleana in Hawaiian culture is ingrained in Kanaka Maoli from a young age—be it duty to family (*'ohana*), community, land, place, or to one's people. The concept of kuleana might end up transforming Hawai'i's food system to benefit all Hawai'i residents.

Similar understandings of the world are found in origin stories from Aotearoa New Zealand, in which the people of the land (*tangata whenua* in Te Reo Māori—the Māori language) were born of Papatūānuku (Earth Mother) and Ranginui (Sky Father), thereby binding the people to nature and its care. This genealogy holds that people are descendants of the natural world and must care for their elders, and to move away from this responsibility is disrespectful and goes against custom. This is clearly a very different understanding of the relationship between nature and humans than the western version(s) with which many readers might be more familiar. In addition, in Aotearoa, women were valued members of their whānau (family). Ani Mikaere states that women "were affirmed and supported throughout their lives. The sharing of work among the whānau (family group) enabled women of child-bearing years to develop their strengths and expertise in a range of areas and to fulfil leadership roles" (2019, 9). The collaborative aspects of their work enabled them to thrive as full-fledged members of their families and within larger tribal associations. The colonizers, however, could not fathom the concept of these women as leaders and, as Tuhiwai Smith (2019) asserts, the Māori internalized the colonizers' perceptions of gender roles, to the long-term detriment of Māori women. Hawai'i and Aotearoa New Zealand present a unique roadmap to resilience and sustainability to draw on as we look for modern solutions through women's stories.

Feminist Political Ecology and Intersectionality

This book uses a feminist political ecology (FPE) framework to structure its argument that women's leadership in AFNs, especially in the context of Oceania, allows us to meaningfully address the problems facing the global industrial agro-food system. FPE is useful in this context because it can be placed in conversation with intersectionality and applied to the settler colonial environments of Oceania. Feminist analysis is integrated within a variety of politico-ecological issues, including sustainable agriculture. As Parker et al. argue, feminist food studies engage with intersectionality to open up "opportunities to deepen our understanding about social inequality and injustice within food systems. Moreover, an intersectional approach demands social change, which we know is needed more than ever given growing social inequalities and concerns about food security and food sovereignty" (2019, 5). Unlike ecofeminism, FPE avoids essentialist constructions of women's roles and draws on political economy and agro-ecological worldviews through the feminist practices of partial perspective and situated knowledges (Haraway 1998; Feldman and Welsh 1995). Ecofeminism's reliance on the biological determinism of women as being closer to nature, especially through the "Mother Earth" metaphor, essentializes women (D'Eaubonne 1974; Griffin 1978; Daly 1978; Shiva and Mies 1993). FPE does not rely on this problematic duality, and instead focuses on understanding the resilience of women's experiences with, and in, the natural world. Lemke and Delormier argue that FPE goes beyond previous feminist analyses by including a political economy approach to uncover the root causes of inequality and power relations (2017). Furthermore, FPE's focus on intersectionality, though imperfect due to its limited focus on race (Mollet and Faria 2013) and indigeneity (Parker et al. 2019), helps to address where marginal identities reside and intersect in order to uncover power dynamics in approaches to food sovereignty. This view clearly supports centering food system inequality as a throughline within intersectional discourse. Indeed, Raj Patel argues that the food sovereignty space has the potential to address deep power inequalities based on sexism, racism, patriarchy, and class power (2013). In fact, a respondent in Stein et al.'s (2018) study of Māori women and community gardens asserted that "self-determination is also leadership" (151). This combination of intersectional situated knowledges and environmental issues also enables the analysis of the neocolonial power dynamics prevalent throughout Oceania.

The wide variety of women's daily lives and experiences are a focus of analysis in FPE. Moreover, understanding "political, economic, cultural and ecological processes as intersectional" (Mulaney 2014, 415) enables us to provide a deeper analysis of women's voices and provide solutions to alternative futures (Rochelau and Nirmal 2014). FPE, especially theoretical interpretations of postcolonial voices, shows women as actors in the ecological and political space, complete with agency and self-determination (Agarwal 1994; Shiva 1988), and values heterogeneity in the lived experiences of women in these ecological spaces (Mohanty 1984), especially in the global South. As Sundberg shows, FPE "demonstrates that political ecological stories are implicated in power relations and researchers risk reproducing gender inequalities if and when women are left out as agents of environmental change" (2017, 8). Indeed, Rochelau et al.'s 1996 edited volume *Feminist Political Ecology* outlines a call for research that analyzes gendered environmental rights and responsibilities, and specifically gendered environmental risks. Following Julier's call to name and practice how we believe we should sustain ourselves and others, we need to do it "loudly and with political power" (2019, 28). I am not simply "adding women and stirring" here to use the often-cited accusation leveled at feminist work. Rather, this book's goal is to ensure that women's voices are front and center.

By paying attention to the ways in which women talk about how gender, race, class, age, and—most importantly—relationships intersect within food systems and the natural world, we make room for their stories to be heard, for their diverse lived experiences of working toward sustainable food systems in various ways to be valued, and for their strength and their work to be celebrated. Turning AFN research on its axis through an intersectional praxis analysis disrupts assumptions about what counts as legitimate food system transformation narratives through epistemological interventions or what Sundberg calls "otherwise neglected dimensions of environmental engagements" (2017, 9). Narratives detailing specific work in community contexts to transform the current food systems that do not serve marginalized peoples help focus our attention on these neglected dimensions. Stories provide the gift of context. So what do these stories tell us about how women are recasting the food system to serve community? How can we apply these lived experiences and concrete actions to a variety of community contexts to improve healthy food access for everyone, not just those with the economic means to purchase healthy foods? How can we value and study Indigenous agricultural systems to rethink our own scientific understanding of sustainable agriculture? How is this work relevant throughout Oceania, yet also applicable in other settler colonial spaces? How does an expansive understanding of intersectional praxis enable us to examine how interlocking systems can work to uplift instead of oppress?

A white western feminist bias would argue that the women in this study are doing the difficult work they are doing because they want to change their respective food systems for their own individual purposes. However, many of the women I talked story with explained that they were involved with these issues because of their roles as mothers, and if the system changed as a result of their work, so much the better. As Leonie Pihama argues in relation to

Māori women, they "live on the cutting edge" (2019, 61). Initially, I thought their gendered responsibilities as mothers would detract from the efficacy and impact of the analysis, but in fact, it seems that my biases got the better of me. In many Indigenous cultures in Oceania, communal responsibility, and responsibility to one's family, broadly defined, is a driving factor for change. Understanding family as community and community as family is part of a larger cultural phenomenon that my own European immigrant background didn't prepare me to recognize as important. *Mana Wāhine Māori*, which exists "irrespective, and often in spite of, the existence of Western feminist networks," helps me address this bias (Pihama 2019, 62). In addition, FPE tries to encompass an intersectional framework that includes an analysis of the impact of colonialism on Indigenous people. It is not my place nor my intention to speak *for* these women, but rather work to amplify their voices in order to show the relationships and connections between their experiences. This bird's-eye view of alternative food system work in Oceania considers these connections to generate food system change. The point is to show how activism around food issues can constitute tangible political achievements and foster a potential political awakening through humility and shared relational experiences and knowledges. It is critical to reflect on the notion of an historic-*ally* honest process—to figure out how to be an ally within a history of dispossession in a settler colonial context, and to actively work to undo centuries of silencing without essentializing Indigenous or marginalized women or communities to deconstruct and unsettle that colonial narrative. In order to support Indigenous women, and all the women doing this important work, this project aims to connect with others to explore stories of successes, challenges, opportunities, difficulties, and joy.

Feminist Food Justice

In neoliberal and neocolonial contexts, feminist food justice has the potential to develop bottom-up approaches to food sovereignty and to reframe what feminist food justice encompasses. Sachs and Patel-Campillo (2014) focus on the scale of agricultural production because, they argue, the smaller the scale, the more likely it is that a woman is making decisions and doing the work, especially those within marginalized racial and ethnic groups. Situating social problems on the micro level (both on the production and the consumption side), however, risks blaming individuals, rather than revealing the "matrix of domination" as defined by Patricia Hill Collins (1990). When our focus remains on micro-level injustices and/or remedies, larger actors such as government, corporations, and supra-national organizations tend to evade scrutiny. Deutsch (2011) argues that a market-based, consumer model relies on individual consumer behavior satisfaction and/or individual producer behavior as a solution, rather than making the necessary overall changes to the food system. Women end up stuck in the middle. Viewing the food system through this neoliberal lens results in an apolitical understanding of the market in which private enterprise and individual consumer behavior are meant to fix a broken food system, without any assistance from the players in control of the structural barriers. Collective action—through movement building within a feminist food justice framework that privileges intersectional analysis and engages in and with postcolonial resistance—is the way to achieve the goals of food system change.

The constant focus on the individual, especially the individual consumer, within our entrenched capitalist culture, is inherently incongruous with food system transformation. We can "vote with our forks" all day long, but until policy and legislative realities value the kind of agriculture that focuses on regenerative practices that leave land and soil better than before, and on implementing sustainable ways of growing and distributing our food, nothing will change. That said, the critique of this consumerist model of social change implicitly means that it is up to the state to legislate and make policy that will incentivize or mandate industry to change its focus away from the profit motive. In the two contexts discussed in this book, the state has not traditionally been a place to turn to for help. In fact, under colonialism, the state has been the entity committing violence against marginalized and Indigenous groups; "indigenous environmental activists coming from the perspective of colonialism tend to be very clear that the state is not an ally" (Norgaard 2019, 160) because, in their view, turning to the state for solutions can have unintended consequences. It is no wonder then, that many groups take matters into their own hands, starting nonprofit groups, businesses, or cooperatives to challenge the industrial agro-food system. Forming and maintaining communities of practice to solve problems can foster feminist food justice in these settler colonial spaces.

It is important to avoid overburdening women with additional roles within AFNs. For instance, Kuo and Peters (2017) found that organic-intensive areas tend to have more women at the helm and are more likely to be embedded within community through CSA programs or direct-to-consumer sales, which may mean additional work for women, even if they are successfully navigating AFNs. The focus of this book goes beyond agricultural production to consider a variety of components that make up AFNs, but likewise relies on women's voices to shape the narrative: community food systems need women to succeed, not only for the women to flourish but for the entire community to reimagine and implement food system change. Kneen (2011) argues that all of these small changes "look innocuous: lots of small initiatives, networked together—in other words, women's work—but [they are] crafting a whole new system, piece by piece" (12). Both the talk story sessions and my engagement with the scholarship demonstrate that these changes alone are not enough and must be coupled with structural change to the food system supported by government and other large players. However, in looking at all of these small actions holistically, we can assess their impact. In fact, the current industrial food system has become so broken that engaging with it through AFNs is not just resistance; it is an act of political engagement. As George McKay writes, "[g]rowing a garden has become—at least potentially—an act of resistance. But it's not simply a gesture of refusal. It's a positive act. It's praxis" (2011, 10). The garden and, on a larger scale, regenerative and sustainable agriculture, are spaces for biodiversity and growth, food system alterity, and justice.

Methods: Talking Story

Snowball sampling was used to recruit participants. I conducted initial talk story sessions with several AFN female leaders, and, at the end of each session, I asked them for names of women who might be willing to participate and have a different perspectives to add to the project. In this way, an initial interview pool of five women leaders in AFNs led to an eventual sample of twenty-nine interviewees in Hawai'i and nineteen interviewees in Aotearoa New Zealand who talked story with me about varying roles in their respective AFNs. The average length of the talk story sessions was about an hour, with one lasting almost three hours and five lasting only thirty minutes. Interviews were recorded using the Voice Memo function on my iPhone, then transcribed using a transcription software service called Trint, checked by me once for accuracy, then provided to each of the respondents to determine whether the transcribed interviews reflected their intent, and finally coded using NVivo 12 software.

In February of 2019, I started casting a wide net for interviewees for this project. I spent some time talking story to twenty-nine women throughout Hawai'i. Although I did not travel to the neighbor islands, and most of the interviews were on O'ahu, I did talk story with several women on Maui, Hawai'i Island,

and Moloka'i, mostly on the phone or using FaceTime. A connection to Kaua'i proved elusive, and I was not able to interview anyone there. I have been teaching a class entitled "Politics of Food" since 2007 that focuses heavily on service-learning. Given this long history of working with a variety of community partners, I formed relationships with many of the people who work to bring about change in the Hawai'i food system. Through this initial access, I was able to ask each interviewee if she could think of anyone else I should speak with in her networks. The women were extremely forthcoming. It is a small, connected community, and each member values her network and what it brings to food system change. The last of these interviews was conducted in February 2020, just prior to my departure for Aotearoa New Zealand. By the time I reached the twentieth or so talk story session, when I asked who else I should interview, quite a few of the names had been mentioned many times and had either already been interviewed or had politely declined. Of the twenty-nine women I interviewed in Hawai'i, seven were Native Hawaiian, eight were local women of color, and fourteen were white. Geographically, twenty-one were based on O'ahu where I live as well, two were on Maui, five were on Hawai'i Island, and one was located on Moloka'i.

The talk story sessions were conducted wherever the interviewees felt comfortable, or it was convenient for them. Several discussions were held at coffee shops or places of work, others on farms, in restaurants, over the phone, over Zoom, or at the respondents' homes. As with any qualitative research, there were interruptions, problems with recordings, and extraneous discussions—about children, families, or common acquaintances. Whenever the occasion presented itself, I purchased the coffee, lunch, or other value-added product being sold by the respondents. I also tried to bring my own agricultural products to share with them, depending on the seasonal availability in my yard—avocados, key limes, starfruit, mangoes, lychee, etc. In other cases, I was encouraged to take as much food as I could carry from a recent harvest and was told in no uncertain terms that I would not be allowed to refuse. The gifts I received were not just material—food to take home to my family—but included knowledge, time, conversation, laughter, kindness, and aloha.

In February 2020, I set out from Auckland in a camper van with a couple of contact names from Gary Maunakea-Forth, co-founder of MA'O Farms on O'ahu, who was born and raised in Aotearoa New Zealand. I drove 1,937 kilometers (about 1,203 miles) in just under three weeks, talking story with women along the way while doing a big loop, first heading north of Auckland, and then south to Wellington on the southern tip of the North Island along the West Coast and then back up the center of the island and briefly to the East Coast. I had already done two video chats with women in Aotearoa New Zealand prior to leaving: one woman was due to deliver a baby very soon and another insisted it would be too far for me to drive to the Far North to interview just her. When I left Hawai'i, I had three guaranteed talk story sessions scheduled. By the time I left Aotearoa New Zealand, I had spoken with fourteen additional women and had two video chats planned for after my return due to scheduling and geographical conflicts. Of the nineteen women I spoke with in Aotearoa New Zealand, all except for one were located on the North Island, eight were Māori, and eleven were white. The number of women—and more importantly the variety among them and the depth of our conversations—went beyond my wildest expectations, thanks largely to one woman whom I came to think of as my fairy godmother of research in Aotearoa New Zealand. Kate Cherrington arranged interviews with key women in the Hua Parakore system along the way. She kept in touch with me every day, making sure I was all right, finding safe places to sleep, helping me gauge routes and distances throughout my trip, and paying for a night's hotel stay in Wellington that had unlimited hot water, a welcome respite from the coin-operated showers I had been taking at all the campgrounds along the way. Without her assistance, this part of the project would never have included the voices of Māori leaders in AFNs and Indigenous food systems. She is a force to be reckoned with in her own right, creating and facilitating countless educational and other programs by and for Māori folks, and ensuring that Māori values are included in other educational and governmental initiatives. Her connections with leading practitioners in Aoetaroa New Zealand's AFNs are what enabled me to avoid the "drop in" researcher dilemma. She helped me foster relationships with women in her networks, and for that I will be forever grateful. Talking story with the Aotearoa New Zealand respondents was transformative for me. I acknowledge this transformation to note how the power of sharing knowledge and experiences through collaborative methodologies increases the feminist objectives of this project.

Before analyzing the data, I sent the raw transcripts (only slightly edited for clarity and 'Ōlelo Hawai'i and Te Reo Māori spelling) to the respondents, asked them if I had correctly transcribed their intent and facts, and if they wanted to provide any edits or make changes. Out of forty-eight respondents, about a quarter took me up on the offer of editing, and eight made significant changes to their narratives. In these cases, I analyzed the updated edited narratives to reflect the ways in which the women wanted to portray their experiences and their work. I considered the interviews separately first, which was useful in its own way, and then compiled them to explore the relationships among the stories. This analysis revealed the major takeaway from this project: although there was some significant overlap in their narratives and motivations, women in two different geographical contexts, with two different colonial oppressors, came up with two different types of responses toward food system transformation. This project positions women as the knowledge holders, not just as agents of change in the moment. They are repositories of stories and hidden meanings, and their willingness to share their work was a significant gift to me and to the research process. Reflecting on their stories fosters inspiration to create connections, networks, and maintain relationships.

My intentional use of qualitative methods, namely culturally appropriate "talk story" sessions with respondents, brings attention to nuances of race, class, ethnicity, and other sociodemographic factors as they may impact gender roles in AFNs and respondents' perception of the problems inherent within the current food system and their ideas for solutions (Stein et al. 2018). Talking story is different than structured or semi-structured interviews because it is rooted in oral history and storytelling traditions throughout Oceania. It is basically akin to chit-chatting and ensuring that all participants feel they are in a safe space to share their *mana'o* (knowledge). In Native Hawaiian and Māori cultures, information and history are passed down to the next generations orally and through stories (Kodama-Nishimoto et al. 1996). This process identifies anyone speaking as a potential teacher and values 'Ōlelo Hawai'i as a language laden with knowledge. Similarly, in Aotearoa New Zealand, one interviewee named Hineāmaru Ropati, a teacher in the Hua Parakore system at the Papatūānuku Kōkiri Marae, explained that she learned through storytelling and through tasting food and physical experiences, which led to her politicization in the food sovereignty space. From a western perspective, Hua Parakore is an Indigenous organic certification program, but from a Māori perspective, it refers to cultural practices that produce food in balance with nature and in turn strengthens Māori cultural practices. Ropati realized that she was looking at the historical journey of Māori in relation to the history and stories of Indigenous peoples everywhere. She asked herself whether Indigenous values existed around the globe. Her answer was that food is the currency with which those values are passed on (Ropati 2020), not only from generation to generation, but are re-learned within the generation that has lost its access to that Indigenous ecological knowledge. This epistemological discovery through storytelling powerfully connects many of the interviewees' narratives. Due to the relatively small sample size, the results of this study are not intended to be generalizable, but they can offer insights into how certain groups of people, in this case women with different racial, class, and geographic identities, may perceive problems, along with their ideas for solutions (Stein et al. 2018). The data do not necessarily fit a predetermined hypothesis and, by respecting and valuing the messiness of the storytelling process, moments of discovery emerge in the women's narratives.

Talking story with the respondents enabled the stories to emerge as a way of honoring the genealogy of the story content and the respondents' work. The stories provided by the interviewees in this project are specific to the food system and not all are from Indigenous sources. Some are from marginalized communities, while other are from women who work with marginalized communities through large educational or health care institutions. Most did see the problematic influence of the colonial legacies in Hawaiʻi and Aotearoa New Zealand—and offered both historical perspectives and solutions to work toward successful and sustainable AFNs. The most important piece of the research paradigm is to ensure cross-dissemination of the research findings and the participants' insights on food system change and alterity in various parts of Oceania. The respondents believe they are obligated to future generations of leaders to learn from failed outcomes and wanted to share their experiences and recognize past mistakes to avoid repeating them. To this end, they all agreed to be identified by name and organization (if applicable) in the book. Identifying the challenges and opportunities faced by different groups of women leaders within AFNs and sharing information among them has the potential to foster new networks of relationality and communication.

Positionality and Practice

Feminist methods commonly focus on women's lived experiences and situated knowledges. Following Allen and Sachs's 2007 call for a feminist food studies, this book expands that focus to the lived experiences of women within AFNs. Intersectional FPE and feminist food justice frameworks intentionally include "analytical power with which to link daily livelihood strategies to broad patterns of inequality and food insecurity. Feminist theory thus provides particularly useful tools with which to tackle the preeminent political question of what kind of natures get produced, how, and by whom" (Mulaney 2014, 408–409). Using Māʻawe Pono, an Indigenous methodological approach developed by Kū Kahakalau (2019), this research maintains attention on building *pono* (righteous) and meaningful relationships among the researcher and the participants of the study. As Kari Marie Norgaard explains of her work in Karuk country, also known as the Klamath Basin in California, "to say that there is an uneasy relationship between tribal communities and academics would be an understatement" (2019, 241). That statement rings just as true for the relationships between Kanaka Maoli, Māori, and academics in Hawai'i and Aotearoa New Zealand respectively. Norgaard (2019) explains that qualitative research in academia tends toward anonymity, but Indigenous peoples *should* be recognized as knowledge holders (instead of research "subjects") and traditional ecological knowledge valued as intellectual property, especially given its potential impact on our future agricultural practices in the face of the climate crisis.

Understanding Mā'awe Pono's impact on data-collection methods is critical to collaboratively finding solutions to current issues and restoring justice to the food system. Kahakalau's methodological framework encourages

> researchers to allow passion, compassion, and comprehension to mingle, the unity of intellect, emotion, and spirit known as lōkahi, becomes transparent... For Hawaiians, the notion of neutrality is incomprehensible, because Hawaiians believe that we bring our mana, or personal power to every situation and every task. This includes all our strengths: physical, emotional, intellectual, and spiritual...In fact, it is this personal mana, or spiritual power, contributed by the researchers to the research process, that gives Mā'awe Pono the power to be a change agent, a beacon of hope for indigenous communities to solve our own problems. (2019, 3)

Using Mā'awe Pono clearly benefits this study and its findings and dovetails with the intersectional praxis perspective of the book. As a (non-Indigenous) researcher, I find it necessary to approach the methodological framework with respect, humility, and grace. In conjunction with feminist methodology, Mā'awe Pono bridges a divide that tends to remain unacknowledged in mainstream feminist literature. Researchers go into certain communities, extract knowledge through interviews with research "subjects," write them up, and get professional/academic credit for the work. No matter how well-intentioned the research projects might be, in settler colonial contexts, this process reproduces the precise extractive practices the research is trying to avoid. Mā'awe Pono's focus on a political commitment to the process of decolonization and the support of Indigenous peoples everywhere (Kahakalau 2019) runs through my research process and imbues my own partial perspective.

This book is a result of research conducted in 2019 and the very beginning of 2020—right before the start of the global COVID-19 pandemic in two geographic locations in Oceania. Further research is needed to determine the pandemic's impacts on the respondents' attitudes toward their roles in their respective food systems. In Hawai'i, where I spent the initial months of self-quarantine and isolation, societal interest in locally grown food grew exponentially during the pandemic. Farm Link Hawai'i, a CSA organization on O'ahu, reported that they provided locally grown produce from around 200 accounts/households per week prior to the pandemic, and grew to 600 accounts per week, with more than 1,500 people on a waiting list that had to be carefully managed so as not to overwhelm their software system (Barreca, personal communication, 2020). Hawai'i imports over 80% of its food (Lyte 2021), whereas Aotearoa New Zealand imports less than 20% (Olsen 2020), simply because there is physical space to grow more food for local consumption and a long-standing ethic of rural living that values working the land that derives from both the Māori and the largely Scottish, English, and Irish early settlers (*Pākehā*) whose descendants now own and work the land. However, much of the land there is geared toward large mono-cropping corporate farms and growing food, especially intensive dairy production, for export. The political response to COVID-19 was different in both places, with Aotearoa New Zealand's prime minister at the time, Jacinda Ardern, closing the country down early in a severe lockdown. Hawai'i followed suit shortly after, though not quite as rigorously. Although this book is not about the effects of the pandemic on the food system, it is worth noting that the pandemic may change our food systems in the long- and short-term—and hopefully for the better.

As Adrienne Rich famously said in 1986, "[b]egin with the material." I want to center and uplift the narratives here, the content of the stories the interviewees were gracious enough to share with me, but also with the material bodies in these stories, which require nourishment of both body and soul. We need good, healthy food to feed ourselves, but the work to get that food into our bodies and those of our families and communities is often taxing and difficult for community and for spirit, though also incredibly rewarding. The Slow Food movement calls this "good, clean, and fair food." The women in this study, and thousands of others in their own communities, make access to this food possible on a daily basis. The implications go beyond individual bodies and reflect changing societal priorities: away from fast, cheap food and toward prioritizing the health of people and the environment.

These processes do not occur in a vacuum. The relationships we make and maintain with our food and with each other are mediated by our own locations (both spatial and metaphorical) within sites of struggle and privilege, and by our access (or lack thereof) to healthcare and wellness, justice, and environments free of pollution and degradation. I started writing this book during what we now know to be a lengthy global pandemic, the height of the Black Lives Matter movement in 2020, and one of the most contentious election years the United States had ever seen. The stakes are high everywhere we look. If we learn anything from these events, it is that without justice, nothing else really matters. Understanding what justice means in different contexts is key: the right not to be killed by police simply for being Black, the rights of Indigenous peoples everywhere to reclaim their ancestral lands and traditions, the rights of people to be free of the various kinds of oppressions they face. I am also writing this as a white, privileged academic woman in Hawai'i, a settler colonial space, who is trying to navigate what it means to be an ally and to constantly renegotiate relationships to support justice and struggles for marginalized people everywhere. Recognizing my privilege, it is my responsibility to use it toward a beneficial purpose and to amplify the voices of women doing the important work of changing their respective food systems. It is certainly not my place, nor my intention, to "speak for others," as Linda Alcoff (1991) has so aptly named this particular problem, but I can use my position of privilege to move the project of reshaping the food system forward.

Getting healthy food to people everywhere while ensuring environmental justice from an intersectional, feminist food justice perspective is not an easy goal to achieve, and it requires a wholesale shift in our systems of food production, distribution, and consumption. The COVID-19 pandemic has taught us that re-localizing our food systems should be a first order priority, especially throughout Oceania. Shipping interruptions threaten the ability to import food to Hawai'i and to export food from Aotearoa New Zealand, with enormous impacts on their respective economies. Hawai'i's incapacity to grow our own food is ill-advised and risky. If mechanisms to import food fail, it is widely reported that Hawai'i only has enough fresh food stored to feed its population for about five days. The figure increases to about ten days if we consider shelf-stable foods (Terrell 2021; McGregor 2018). Currently, the centralized food system—owned and operated by industrial-agriculture capitalists through agglomerated multinational corporations—is doing communities everywhere a disservice. This is nothing new, but it is worth noting that during the pandemic, many people had the time to think about where their food comes from and to consider whether they have the capacity to grow and cook it themselves. At the height of quarantine in 2020, I learned from an emergency trip to a chain hardware store that there was no packaged soil available on the island of O'ahu, and I was told that there would be none for the foreseeable future. So many people were trying to learn to grow their own food that they had bought all of the soil. People took this time to learn about growing food for their own consumption or about supporting their local farmers through home deliveries of CSA boxes. These are huge steps toward lessening our dependency on imported foods. However, this context of the "new normal" of pandemic living was by definition temporary, and we must figure out how to maintain this interest in the long term. Institutional and government support will be key to sustaining these positive changes through just and equitable means.

Telling someone else's story implies one has some kind of power over it—that of the omniscient researcher, interpreting someone else's tale. However, the point here is power *with*, not power *over*. I have been partially embedded in (some of) these worlds for almost two decades, and through those relationships and associations, I discovered new (to me) spaces wherein women are doing interesting and different work in and around the food system. Meeting in informal settings enabled us to come together to share stories and to exchange experiences and knowledge. I am *in* the research, *in* the narrative, either because our experiences are somewhat familiar or because we discover we have common bonds—children of the same age, similar interests outside of work, curiosity about growing certain crops, or even a shared appreciation for certain kinds of foods. My presence as an interviewer is perceptible in the stories. Although I asked no specific questions and didn't have a structured or even unstructured interview schedule, I did ask all the participants to tell me about their work. In her work on the partition of India, Butalia quotes Roland Barthes and says she is suspicious of what Barthes calls stories that "seem to write themselves" (2000, 15). Likewise, it is not my intention to make it seem like these stories came out of nowhere. They are political statements on the status quo of the current food system as much as they show a commitment to changing it—both on the part of the respondents and myself. I cannot remove myself from the discussion; indeed, I have no plans to do so. Clearly, there is intention behind soliciting these stories, just as there is intention behind asking specific people to share them. The stories themselves are not objective, nor do their tellers purport to be. The point is to center the women telling these stories and their work in food system change. It is not about "giving" them voice—their voices have been there—but about making sure we listen to what they are saying by making space for those voices to be heard. Although I provide interpretation and analysis of the narratives presented, I do so *alongside* the voices of the women talking story. My analysis certainly does not supersede the stories; rather, the goal is to enhance them by highlighting their connections and to enable an intersectional feminist interpretation of the nuanced experiences of women within food systems in Oceania to come to the fore.

Telling someone else's story can also be akin to taking it and making it one's own. It is not my intention to reproduce the colonizing effects of taking what's not mine. Rather, my intent is to amplify the stories and tell them *with* the interviewees, to disseminate their knowledge to that others may replicate their successes and learn from their challenges. Butalia calls the implications of this work as revealing the "broader political realities" (2000, 71). She is referring to the stories of India's partition from the perspective of "bit players," but her focus on small stories within the context of larger political and social movements is similar to this book's intent. I attempt to weave together stories and the politics of food systems change within neocolonial contexts in Oceania by centering the stories instead of the grand political gestures and frequently meaningless rhetoric around greenwashed local food production. This work asks, how do real people effect real food system change? How can we learn from them and each other? How does this work—which is so often seen as "women's work" because it relates to food until it becomes more public through (mostly male) chefs and/or politicians—affect society at large? Listening to women's voices enables us to focus on the implications of this work on real people, rather than talking about contexts and obstacles so large that they seem insurmountable.

This project is a necessary first step toward creating networks of relationships in food systems across Oceania. What works in one geographic, political, and neocolonial context may not necessarily work in another, but there are lessons to be learned through the stories told. These stories reflect the future food systems we want to see and work toward, not just the current political context of our respective food systems. That future will enable us to create food systems that work for everyone, regardless of gender, race, class, ethnicity, or geographic location. Focusing on women's voices shows that women are among the most dedicated in doing the work of food system change, but also tend to be among the most affected by broken food systems everywhere.

Food Stories as Counterdiscourse

This project advances a new vision of feminist food studies (Allen and Sachs 2007; Avakian and Haber 2006) and responds particularly to Kimura's suggestion that a feminist reading of women's leadership in alternative food networks holds AFNs "accountable for [their] social justice implications and distributive effects" (Kimura 2012, 211). This intersectional approach to food systems stretches the narratives around AFNs to include women's voices and shared wisdom and contributes to tending the soil and the bodies and minds of community. Nancy Fraser refers to the role of "counterpublics...to invent and circulate counterdiscourses...and to help expand discursive spaces" (1990, 67). Paying attention to

the role of intersectionality in the respondents' stories broadens our understanding of the food systems in Hawaiʻi and Aotearoa and highlights the multiple modes of subordination currently present in the industrialized agro-food system. The path forward depends on increased participation in and leadership by women in community-based food systems. This is made clear by both the similarities and differences between Hawaiʻi and Aotearoa; thus, the chapters are organized thematically, not geographically, in order to highlight the connections among the stories' perspectives. Both spaces—colonized by the United States and the British empires respectively—indicate that regardless of the trajectory of response, resistance within the food system requires centering not just gender, but race, class, and indigeneity, among other socially constructed realities. It is not enough for food system activists to encourage individuals to make changes in their consumption patterns; rather, it is imperative to contextualize food system transformation through the diverse experiences of women working and living within AFNs. These responses have been shaped by neocolonial processes in different ways, and there are spaces of both oppression and privilege within AFNs. Norgaard (2019) articulated that academia, and the discipline of sociology in particular, does a disservice to Native communities by ignoring their voices and their centuries of experiences with nature and ecological practices, based on Indigenous scientific knowledge passed down through generations. Moreover, she identifies a lack of "the sociological imagination" as one reason for this oversight. In the chapters that follow, I call for the *political imagination* to embrace these voices and uplift these experiences as pragmatic solutions to the problems we face in our food systems and related issues like climate change. Ignoring Native voices does not just do a disservice to Native communities but leaves us less capable of understanding the modern moment, because we exclude voices that already have answers to the questions we are asking—and have likely had these answers for centuries.

Intersectional praxis within FPE enables an understanding of varied settler colonial contexts and the ways different groups negotiate and respond to the ongoing violence of the colonial project that continues to separate agriculture from community. The grounded theory emerging from the narratives demonstrates the application of themes and concepts through relational intersectional perspectives, which Collins and Bilge (2020) indicate as a desirable outcome for burgeoning social justice movements. Anti-colonialism actively resists the neocolonial project and its sustained marginalization of certain groups of people. The anti-colonial project is not *just* about reclaiming land in a larger Land Back movement as outlined by Indigenous peoples everywhere seeking not only to secure land, but also pushing for self-determination, environmental sustainability, and economic viability to build "collective power and collective liberation" (Belfi and Sandiford 2021). The Red Nation's *Red New Deal* states that "having control over our ancestral territories is vital to our ability to care for them and is a generations-long pathway to true sustainability. Only when land is restored and returned, can we begin to rebuild our economies and our nations with true sovereignty" (2021). This project aims to center that work in both Hawai'i and Aotearoa New Zealand, as it also requires forming, strengthening, and maintaining community relationships and increasing the focus on acknowledging and resisting the colonial processes embedded within our everyday lives.

Land is a part of Indigenous communities' connections with their ancestors, and responsibility for and kinship to land form a crucial set of networked relationships that create community in the first place. The potential for food system change occurs when agency expresses resistance. The question is, which acts of resistance best benefit the larger community? Reinvigorating Indigenous values about the importance of land as it relates to genealogy is one of these very powerful measures. This esteem is typically community held, and its attrition in the neocolonial context weakens a community's bond to the land and, by extension, its community members. Communities that focus on renewing these Indigenous values have begun to reestablish community-led food sovereignty, as in the case of MA'O Farms on the Leeward Coast of O'ahu, for example, or the different Hua Parakore spaces in Aotearoa. Counterdiscourses to unequal access to good, clean, and fair food rise up within these spaces to challenge the global industrialized agro-food system in order to serve marginalized communities. Although Daniel Immerwahr argues that "empire is held not by taking over land, but by the market" (2019, 315), the capitalist system has cemented itself in place by taking over both land and market and creating neocolonial spaces everywhere. Given my argument for centering gender and other socially constructed realities, it is not surprising that ensuring forward momentum appears to fall on the backs of women. However, adding yet another load to women's work is not the goal of this project. I argue that it is instead imperative to understand how these spaces have created openings for resistance and opportunities to disrupt a monolithic capitalist system intent on crushing any opposition to its intrinsic goals of domination. This is key to changing the current state of the global industrial agro-food system.

Themes and Chapter Overviews

This book is organized thematically to showcase the stories of women working toward food system transformation in Hawai'i and Aotearoa New Zealand. Instead of using a comparative geographic perspective to organize the book, I chose to weave distinct themes I identified in the stories within each chapter, going back and forth between Hawai'i and Aotearoa New Zealand depending on where the stories led me. Chapters 1 and 2 establish how land-use policy affects the food system in each context. Then, Chapters 3, 4, and 5 each focus in on a distinct theme. In Chapter 6, I take a step back and undertake a comparative analysis of community engagement within food systems at work in each place. Each chapter moves between narratives from Hawai'i and Aotearoa New Zealand, such that connections and differences between these two contexts emerge.

More specifically, Chapter 1 addresses environmental components of sustainable agriculture through the lens of decolonizing agriculture and food systems in Oceania. Land-use zoning and the pressures of the housing development industry in Hawai'i have set up a battle for the future of land and the potential for sustainable regional community food systems. In Aotearoa New Zealand, conventional farming constitutes a large majority of the agricultural sector, both for local consumption and for export. There are, of course, plenty of organic farmers, as well as people focused on regenerative and agroecological practices to feed their families and communities. Indeed, they co-constitute the AFN movement in Aotearoa New Zealand. If there is any chance for food sovereignty in the context of the climate crisis in the island environments of Hawai'i or Aotearoa New Zealand, regenerative and sustainable agriculture must become priorities. Policy and legislative practice's continued focus on the settler colonial model of large plantation agriculture is a detriment to food system transformation. Although the land scarcity model is less pronounced in Aotearoa than it is in Hawai'i, the fact that many Kanaka Maoli and Māori people still do not have access to land reinforces the neocolonial relationship that Indigenous peoples have with their respective settler colonial states. In both cases, the genealogy of Indigenous people is tied to the land, and acknowledging the violence done to their ancestors—including the theft of the land itself, appropriation, commodification, and industrialized agriculture—would allow everyone to take a step back and listen to the stories and voices of women working in this space to implement change.

Chapter 2 uses the lens of traditional ecological knowledge and Indigenous agricultural systems to narrow the focus on the relationship between land and environment. I highlight a particular emphasis on stewardship and natural resource management and consider how an intersectional approach supports the argument for combining Indigenous and traditional farming practices. The soils of Hawai'i and Aotearoa New Zealand have been depleted by decades of intensive industrial mono-cropping. Nourishing the soil means nourishing people and reconceptualizing our understanding of the importance of regenerating soils to foster sustainable agriculture and what it means to environmental health and justice is key.

Chapter 3 examines the relationship between education and social justice within the food system in Hawai'i and Aotearoa New Zealand. Hawai'i's focus on educating children through farm-to-school programs is not unique, and there are many similar efforts underway on the continent through the Department of Education and a multitude of nonprofit organizations. The farm-to-school emphasis is not nearly as pronounced in Aotearoa New Zealand, and nonprofit organizations are essentially missing from the conversation surrounding food systems transformation there. Instead, for example, the Hua Parakore organization's focus is on education, especially of Māori women, to take information and skills about culturally appropriate gardening and cooking home to their families and communities—that is, to use Māori culture as a way to address food system injustices and access. Māori knowledge passed down from generations about sustainable agriculture is being woven into a variety of programs to disseminate information about the value of traditional ecological knowledge and its importance in combating climate change. Through hard work based on exhaustive qualitative research by educators there, Māori culture is being included in the educational system to the extent that a system of culturally-based educational centers has been created to focus on regenerating the Māori food system in service to both Māori communities and society at large. The idea is that the more people know how to grow their own culturally appropriate food, the less dependent they will be on take-out shops and fast food options for their nutritional intake. Even non-Māori descendants of European settler Pākehā women who work in this field take the Māori worldview of sustainable agriculture and connectedness with nature into account in their programs and narratives.

Chapter 4 focuses on public and community nutrition and health by examining culturally appropriate foods as a way to pursue food sovereignty and the public health impacts of decolonizing our diets. There are clearly connections between good nutrition and sustainable environmental practices. This chapter views these connections through the lens of cultural identity, which identifies food as culture. I examine school lunch programs in several ways: as educational spaces for children to understand the importance of healthy local foods in their diets; as examples of gendered attitudes toward cooking and its relationship to public, community, and family health; and as spaces where the state, through its administration of programs, can promote food system transformation. To supplement the analysis of school lunch, this chapter examines the connection between nutrition, environmental sustainability, and food as a crucial component of cultural identity.

Chapter 5 raises questions about sustainable meat- and fish-derived protein production and consumption through an intersectional lens, interrogating how gender, race, and class, among other analytic categories, interact to create spaces for women to engage with what has traditionally been considered masculine work, such as dairying, fishing, ranching, and butchering. These alternative (rather than industrial) efforts to produce and consume protein (meat, fish, and dairy) in Hawai'i and Aotearoa New Zealand are exemplary in that they occur in closed ecosystems and use innovative models to address environmental issues such as invasive species like axis deer, overfishing, and sustainable dairy production. This chapter considers these components of diets in relation to the gendered (and raced, and classed) aspects of other diet options, such as vegan or vegetarian diets, which are themselves often part of AFNs.

Chapter 6 shows the relationships and emergent themes in stories from the two separate geographic contexts and examines how they can enhance and support each other. Although there are clear differences and variations, likely due to the different colonial contexts as well as the political and societal values in each space, the similarities are striking and worthy of attention. This chapter identifies policy implications for each location, and highlights women's leadership roles in pushing for food system transformation through community engagement.

A running theme throughout the narratives challenges the standard definition of "success" within the global capitalist system. The respondents offer alternatives and explain how to foster food system resilience in the face of the climate crisis. The takeaways from this project have the potential to help us change our food systems for the benefit of all.

CHAPTER 1

Decolonizing Agriculture and Food Systems

He Wahine, He Whenua—E Ora ai te Iwi / By Women and Land, People are Sustained.
—Ripeka Evans (2019)

'*Āina* and *Whenua* As/Is Family

Genealogically, in both Kanaka Maoli and Māori worldviews, land is considered the people's ancestor. Different cosmologies are associated with this relationship, but common to all is the view that one does not harm the land since it is part of one's family. The extractive capitalist agricultural model simply does not fit within this perspective. Despite the nuances in the creation stories they mentioned, many of the interviewees reflected similar beliefs about the relationships between humans, land, and different parts of the ecosystem. In western terms, this could also encompass an agroecological view of the relationship between land and humans, although the latter does not include a kinship or spiritual relationship and is necessarily different in that regard. Prior to arriving in Auckland in 2020, I spoke via Zoom with Rangimārie Mules, co-director of the Oi Collective, a group of women who lead social innovation and community-building efforts around Aotearoa New Zealand. She offered a postcolonial feminist interpretation of the Māori creation story:

> Within our own cultural revitalization, the female stories are emerging. We were brought up knowing that the first human was a woman, and she was made from the sands of mother earth. And her offspring was in this world, but then moved into the underworld to be the person to welcome people into the afterlife. Rather than being the maiden of the night, the postcolonial feminist narrative around her is that she's actually the first voice for the spirits of the afterlife. It's a lot more of a positive thing than some of the other kind of narratives which are around

her being condemned to that area. The process by which she made that choice was hers. As females, it's about making the choice under certain circumstances, and we've got that ability. I just think in terms of our culture, there is a deeper motivation. That's the connection that comes from our bones. It's from our genealogical point of reference. It's just this innate thing from a Māori perspective that connects woman and land. (Mules 2020)

Mules's explanation of Māori cosmology identifies women's role as central to Māori society. Indeed, Māori stories share the importance of women in Māori culture through the naming of hapū (subtribes or kinship groups) after women in many iwi tribes (Mikaere 2019), for example, or through an analysis of Te Reo Māori, which utilizes gender-neutral pronouns. Colonizers did not have the capacity to understand women's roles as leaders and thus erased their stories from the colonized reality.

Mules's narrative shows the connectedness of Māori wisdom between past, present, and future as it relates to land and to growing food through a central Māori creation story that highlights powerful women:

The whenua, the placenta that you grow and birth, is also the same word for land. I think it's a human story that weaves all of that together, which is around our ability to endure. Coming from an Indigenous lens, so many things set you up to be motivated to be an active person in terms of environmental interaction. *And it has to be intertwined with cultural revitalization, because if we don't, we lose all of that richness, and all of that motivation and intention and we become gardeners of the surface landscape, not gardeners of hope, of society.* And when we talk about food systems, it has to be a closed loop system. It has to be value added. That has to be all of those things that allow cycles to go, go, go, systems to go, go, resilience and adaptation, all of that, to move in, and be fluid. If we just become workers of the surface, gardeners of the surface of the landscape then we'll just die out and get pushed out. We have a deeper notion of why we do things. (Mules 2020, emphasis added)

Of all the women I interviewed, Mules provides one of the most meaningful explanations of the importance of kinship and spiritual connections between land and Indigenous peoples. Her stories reflect the depth of understanding that she has about how her indigeneity—her Māori-ness—helps her recognize that humans and ecosystems are connected. This shows how intersectional praxis in

FPE reflects Indigenous understandings of the connection between land and people and leads to adaptability and resilience. At the same time, however, Mules's reflection begs the following questions: Why should women have to do *more* work? Why should they be *more* resilient? Why should they be *more* steadfast in their commitment to intersectional justice in AFNs—especially, if this work is being done by Indigenous women all over the world? The short answer is they *shouldn't have* to do or be any of those things, but they do anyway. Because no one else is doing it. They are stepping up to fix the broken food system.

This undercurrent runs through many of the narratives, although it manifests in different ways: families are not necessarily nuclear in nature, and certainly not in Māori nor in Kanaka Maoli cultures, which value collective child rearing. Nor are communities bound by geographic borders. Rather, they are families and communities of shared ideas, shared values, and even shared foods. But as Lehn Huff, the director of the Maui School Garden Network reminds us,

> In the context of oral history, which then becomes a written history, we lose the power of women. I'm going to hold on to that thought because we're talking about women in farming....We're connected to the land. Why do civilizations fail? A lot of that had to do with the relationship to the land, not using the land appropriately.
>
> The majority of people I work with statewide and locally are women. I work with a lot of great young men and women of all ages. But I'm just saying, the majority is definitely women. Maybe it is because it's connected to education. You tend to find more women in education, right? When you get close to the earth, we always think of it as Mother Earth. But I would also say women are getting more into leadership roles now. I see women going out there and helping to create and manage food hubs, distribution centers like that center on the Big Island. (Huff 2019)

Women's leadership enables more women to thrive in this political space. This work is difficult and often poorly remunerated, likely because it is traditionally associated with women. Betsy Cole, the former program director at the Kohala Center, an independent, community-based nonprofit focused on research, education, and ʻāina stewardship for healthier ecosystems, shares:

> I'm thinking in terms of interest in local food systems, regenerative agriculture, although there are men doing the work, including running farms, but the systemic work does also seem to be the role of women right now. And of course, there's no money in it.

> I know that's a little bit glib. So that's part of it, men really have more pressure, not that they are necessarily the breadwinners anymore. But it's an orientation toward what kind of success, in an American capitalist society, that you need to have. (Cole 2019)

Here, Cole highlights the connections between the American capitalist definition of success, the roles of women, value systems, education, mothering and feeding children, through the lens of neocolonialism in Hawai'i. She goes on to focus on gender roles throughout the colonization process. She argues that men stand to lose more in a disruption of the status quo because colonizing forces granted them more rights than women through patriarchal legal frameworks rooted in western jurisprudence.

> But it always seemed to me that women were less placed in dysphoria by colonization because they still had a role in childbirth and family still had that sort of a primary role. That didn't change. But for men, when a culture is disrupted, their roles get disrupted more on some level. Their power structure gets taken away and it's a much larger drop. If you translate the amount of power that they still have, you're not left with any role. Whereas women still have a sense of purpose. (Cole 2019)

Cole's words resonate with Gayatri Chakravorty Spivak's formulation of strategic essentialism (Spivak 1985), which she conceives as a provisional acceptance of essentialist identity categories as a political tactic to mobilize in struggle. Women's roles within families are central to their power in both Kanaka Maoli and Māori cultures, yet were reformulated by colonizers to be worth less than the roles of men. Cole, along with several other respondents, mentions women's gendered roles as mothers and caregivers as central to both their identities and reasons for being involved with food system change. Using strategic essentialism to critique women's roles as mothers and other caregiving roles has the potential to dismantle the existing food system through political intentionality, but it skirts dangerous territory. Using it can lead us to uncritically rely on the "as women" trope, jettisoning not only intersectional analysis, but flattening women's lived experiences in AFNs. It is critical to avoid reducing women's roles or Native Peoples to single identities. Are they mothers or educators? Or both? Are they from urban or rural areas? Are they from particular kinship groups? Particular geographic regions? Do they have specific political ideologies? What are their gendered, raced, and/or classed relationships to land? Valuing heterogeneity in gender and Indigenous identities and their respective knowledges helps remedy the epistemic violence done by decades of western ideas imposed on the food system. Cole's decades of leadership at the Kohala Center on Hawai'i Island helped her see women's roles in the alternative food movement from a more holistic perspective. This complexity results from the many roles women perform in their daily lives. It is also representative of the multiplicity of roles available to women within the sustainable food system community. Ka'iulani Oddom, the Roots Program director at the Kōkua Kalihi Valley Community Health Center, a land-based nutrition program, also finds that "relationships and everything we do are more important than statistics. They're more important than money. They're more important than anything else. It's about making sure that our relationships are solid and that we're respectful of each other" (Oddom 2019). Indeed, family and community have been a constant source of strength for many of the respondents interviewed for this book.

Geographic Contexts

Located around 2,500 miles from the continental United States, Hawai'i is the most geographically isolated land mass in the world. Yet the archipelago is a part of what has been called the Polynesian Triangle[1] and it is connected with much of Oceania through migration as well as geographic and cultural similarities. Islands are both microcosms and accelerators of knowledge; due to their isolation, they enable inhabitants to observe and develop knowledge of various kinds, especially in the natural sciences, relying on Indigenous knowledge of plants, animals, flora, and fauna. As is often touted in this age of climate change, two-thirds of the planet is made up of oceans and the islands within them; however, although they are separated by water, islands are not isolated. They are often grouped in archipelagos, connected to each other or to distant metropolises, and are linked through the movement of goods, people, and cultural practices. Islands are connected to the rest of the world and its material flows. Referring to Oceania, Epeli Hau'ofa has famously called this phenomenon "our sea of islands" (1994). In Polynesian stories, a mythical place called Hawaiki is the starting point of migration between Polynesian spaces, although it is not clear which of the geographical areas is meant by the moniker. This origin story is found in both Māori creation stories

---

[1.] The term "Polynesia" is problematic because it indicates the separation of Pacific peoples into different groups by European explorers. The 'Ōlelo Hawai'i term Moananuiākea is an alternative term meaning great expansive ocean. It encompasses a myriad of Indigenous peoples who are connected genealogically.

and Kanaka Maoli worldviews, among others throughout Oceania. Appreciating island connectedness helps us understand why Hawai'i's and Aotearoa New Zealand's food systems are relevant to the entire Pacific region.

Given Hawai'i's place as the fiftieth state in the US, Native Hawaiian culture is often commodified and objectified, especially in the service of ever-increasing tourism dollars. Haunani-Kay Trask famously condemned the islands' commodification of Native Hawaiian culture in her 1991 article "Lovely Hula Hands." The food system is defined by the multinational corporations omnipresent in Hawai'i, such as fast food companies, grocery, super store chains, and convenience stores. These serve to make the unfamiliar familiar to an exceedingly large number of tourists—approximately 10 million in 2019 and, after the travel restrictions during the pandemic, this number resumed in 2025 and beyond. After all, people might visit Hawai'i for its physical beauty, but also because all of the comforts of "home" are present as well. The same is true for the large military population of people from all over the contiguous US who are used to having all of the conveniences of home at their fingertips. The food system in Hawai'i embodies distance, but with some familiarity. Although the McDonald's in Hawai'i serves the same Big Mac as a McDonald's on the continent, it also serves Portuguese sausage for breakfast and taro pies for dessert. It's the same, but with a little twist; different yet familiar. Indeed, McDonald's has different "local" items on menus globally. Multinational corporations embody the newer version of colonizers, structured to optimize their own wealth instead of community health. Once again, culture is commodified to increase profits. In addition, with fast food, women are blamed for opting to rely on the kind of convenience food that is constantly marketed to them as an easy and cheap way to feed their families. An intersectional FPE framework is capable of overturning this narrative by doing the work of understanding how the food system can be deconstructed and rebuilt to recognize the work of women, and more specifically women of color, Indigenous women, or women from marginalized communities within this sector, not just as consumers, but as agents of change.

Aotearoa New Zealand is the southernmost point of the Polynesian Triangle, as problematic as that term may be, and is surrounded by the Pacific Ocean on three sides and the Tasman Sea on the West side stretching toward Australia. It mainly consists of two large islands—the North and South Islands—or Te Ika-a-Māui and Te Waipounamu in Te Reo Māori respectively. The islands contain a multitude of climates and geographic features like mountainous terrain, rolling hills, sandy beaches, rocky shorelines, and very deep fjords. It is an incredibly scenic and biodiverse landmass. In Aotearoa New Zealand, Māori culture is quite prevalent, and is both respected and consulted on numerous issues, with laws and policies codified in government structures that require frequent consultation with Māori folks on issues related to land, water, and Māori culture. That said, several respondents indicated that the reality is often different from the stated policies. Nevertheless, the fact that there are structural processes in place stemming from the Treaty of Waitangi/Te Tiriti O Waitangi, however questionable that may have been, means that Māori culture and tribes are at minimum legally recognized. In Aotearoa New Zealand, rural places don't have the same kind of multinational corporate pressure to open their communities to fast-food and convenience store chains. This is not to say that there is no fast food—there is indeed. Takeaway shops with fried foods and meat pies are prevalent in many areas, no matter the socioeconomic status and demographics of the community. Indeed, at those shops, one can get a calorie-dense, if nutritionally deficient, meal for a very reasonable NZ$8 to NZ$11. Converted to USD (2025) —that is, between $6 USD and $8 USD—an extremely cheap and fast meal. Although the food will likely be fried and wrapped in butcher paper or Styrofoam, these takeaway shops are not generally owned by multinational corporations.

Decolonizing Food Systems

The women I interviewed in Aotearoa New Zealand were much more explicit in their attention to colonization's effects on the food system than were the women in Hawai'i, and more focused on *de*colonizing processes through existing legal structures and contexts. Although they work within the system, the system inherently makes room for Māori voices and programs to resonate and engage society, not necessarily because it wants to, but because it has to, legally. Shirley (2013) argues that Te Tiriti O Waitangi, the founding document of the colonial relationship between Aotearoa New Zealand and the British, was supposed to be translated verbatim into English as the Treaty of Waitangi—a document of peace and friendship. This was supposed to give Māori legal recognition and a voice and role within government. However, the English version (Treaty of Waitangi) ceded Māori sovereignty to the Crown and justified the colonization of Aotearoa New Zealand by the British. Both versions were signed by the Māori, with disastrous consequences for Māori culture and Indigenous land dispossession. Narratives of colonialism are much more prevalent in the literature on the Māori food system than elsewhere precisely because of the intentional mistranslation of Te Tiriti O Waitangi into English. It outlines the concept of land ownership, now clearly defined, and used as a basis for legal arguments and settlements. The injustices of Māori land dispossession through colonization then, are much more apparent in the Aotearoa New Zealand narratives than they were in Hawai'i. The legal system's acknowledgment of Māori rights due to the existence of Te Tiriti O Waitangi means that there is much more room to maneuver to successfully fight colonial occupation in Aotearoa New Zealand, though there is always a danger that a top-down approach might not be ideal, nor successful in the long term.

Given this politico-legal framework, food sovereignty inherently resists colonization because it places the food system of Aotearoa New Zealand in an historical context—and long-standing interactions with the British are relevant on a daily basis due to an export agriculture economy based on neoliberal capitalist principles. The academic literature contradicts itself in terms of Aotearoa New Zealand's food sovereignty overall. Stevenson (2011) argues that there is enough food grown in Aotearoa New Zealand, but Bartos (2016) argues that although there is plenty of food grown in the nation, most of it is exported, a practice that maintains and reinforces the colonial history of growing food for export to Britain. For example, the dairy industry, which constitutes about one-third of the entire global trade in dairy, exports nearly 95% of its milk production (Dairy Companies Association of New Zealand 2020), mostly to China in order to make reconstituted milk and baby formula. This type of export-oriented food system fundamentally separates people from land and from their genealogies. Ngahuia Te Awekotuku cites Linda Tuhiwai Smith's assertion that "by just being Māori and a woman who thinks about her life, and her people—one is on the cutting edge. That is where Māori women live—on the cutting edge of theory. And that edge cuts deep, sharpened by our experience as a post-colonial people" (1991, 24–25).

Food was used as a tool for colonization as much as it is being used now as a tool for resistance. Kate Cherrington, chair of Te Pūtea Whakatupu Trust (now renamed Tapuwae Roa), an organization dedicated to the sustenance of Māori identity through various projects, especially those related to whenua (land), whānau (family), and Indigenous ways of knowing, explained precisely how food became almost a bludgeon in the service of colonizing practices:

> You know, around food sovereignty, around self-determining food systems, what's enough may be enough for sharing with a neighbor. What I get, it would be for all. It could be for others, not for me to stockpile. If you think about it, there was no refrigeration in ancient times, so it's like you couldn't stockpile, you had to share right away. Refrigeration and being able to transport things is

part of the colonial story, right. It's being able to transport things to England, refrigerate, and drive. And we were right there as the colonial outpost, sending our sheep. (Cherrington 2020)

She explains how Aotearoa New Zealand was complicit in its own colonization and how Indigenous food system practices of sharing and gifting were quickly eroded to make way for a profit motive-based export agriculture. Refrigeration technology was just as important in Hawai'i, where the dependence on imported foods was clearly aided by refrigerated container ships that were able to provide cheaper food products from the continent than could be grown in Hawai'i due to high land and labor costs. These roadblocks to a healthy food system are still firmly entrenched in both places. Furthermore, refrigeration and the long journeys of exported foods in both instances affect nutritional value. When it is picked early and stored for weeks, or in some cases even months, the nutrient content of food decreases over time, so the food received on either end is neither fresh, nor nutritionally dense.

Colonization and Agricultural History/Colonial Legacies

How did Hawai'i arrive at a wholly dependent food system and Aotearoa New Zealand arrive at an export-driven food system? The ongoing processes of colonization are responsible in both cases: marginalizing Native Hawaiians and Māori, leading to the dispossession of their land, and creating the conditions for a land-use policy in the early and mid-nineteenth century that facilitated the purchase of large tracts of land by agribusiness corporations. In Hawai'i, these landowners initially produced sugarcane and pineapple for export using workers imported primarily from Asia to labor in the fields. Once it became apparent that these two tropical crops could be grown more cheaply by exploiting workers in the global South, the plantations shuttered in service of neocolonial policies elsewhere. Under the guise of "globalization," the International Monetary Fund's (IMF) structural adjustment policies created conditions whereby brown people beyond Hawai'i's shores were forced to work for low wages to farm crops for export to developed nations. The players may have changed, but the situation remains the same. In Aotearoa New Zealand, land is also concentrated in the hands of a few corporations, but due to treaty obligations toward Māori people, several iwi do have control over large tracts of land. There are also many Pākehā (white, settler) landowners of medium-sized farms, who are either descendants of immigrants from Britain during the nineteenth century or Pākehā veterans who were given land upon returning from World War II. Land was not given to returning Māori veterans however, exacerbating the colonizing forces of land dispossession even late into the twentieth century.

In both places, agricultural lands are concentrated in the hands of few owners. In Hawai'i, because agricultural production remains prohibitively expensive, much of the land is either fallow or is used for genetically modified crop experiments by large chemical companies. The end result is that Hawai'i grows very little of its own food, although interest in reducing that dependence on imported food has increased (Costa and Besio 2011). The reality is that the colonial power relations that produced this situation remain firmly entrenched. Indeed, the neoliberal market conditions that encourage a focus on cheap food reinscribe the colonial project. Daniel Immerwahr (2019) argues that "[t]he great coordinating process isn't colonial rule, which operates within borders, but globalization, which crosses them" (315). Nothing could be more accurate in the case of Hawai'i and Aotearoa New Zealand. The American and British exploitation of Kanaka Maoli and Māori notions of land stewardship, respectively, through land privatization that reinforced western notions of land ownership meant—and continues to mean—that Native Hawaiian and Māori lands were stolen from them during and after the *māhele* (land division) of 1848 and after the signing of the Treaty of Waitangi in 1840. Kanaka Maoli and Māori worldviews are based on familial relationships to land, resulting in a gifting economy. The land provides sustenance because it is itself, family. This signifies a completely different view of the relationship to land than what might exist in a western conception.

Manifest Destiny dictated the "inevitability" of territorial expansion, fueled by imperialist desires, and resulted in an extractive worldview of nature. This eventually resulted in the conditions by which large tracts of land were aggregated and purchased by a small number of owners. Current market conditions and land-use policies exacerbate the situation. Agricultural land is prohibitively expensive, especially because it is not available in small parcels, creating almost insurmountable barriers to entry for new farmers. In Hawai'i, the result is a continued dependence on imported foods and the precarious food system's sustained lack of resilience in the face of worsening climate change. In Aotearoa New Zealand, large conventional farms continue to monocrop for export, dwarfing any meaningful attempt to create AFNs. Emily King (2020), the director of Spira NZ, an organization focused on building resilience and sustainability of food systems based on New Zealand's North Island, explained:

We have agricultural strategies because we have an unusually strong agricultural sector with large-scale dairy farms. We have irrigation issues because what we've done is basically created large areas of dry toxic land that was once frozen in the forest and converted into irrigated farms in the South Island particularly. There are these massive water allocation issues and stress on catchments. We have a lot of stream pollution directly resulting from runoff. And that's a sore point with consumers and generally environments and pollution. There is a whole regenerative agriculture movement right now with lots of farmers changing our best practices, but the movement is still very small. (King 2020)

Here, King explains that large-scale, export-focused industrial agriculture in Aotearoa New Zealand has polluted land and water, although there are efforts to move toward more sustainable agricultural practices, even if they are only in the early stages. Additionally, the ongoing neocolonial project means that the descendants of both white missionary-turned-capitalist land barons and of the laborers who were imported earlier are now leaders of industry, development, and politics. As Norgaard argues, "the supposed innocence of settlers in this process was upheld by claims of inevitability, the discourse of progress and human evolution, and racialized notions of Native inferiority" (2019, 53). This feigned innocence obscures the reality of continued land dispossession of Kanaka Maoli, Māori, and other marginalized communities in both places, namely Pasifika immigrants and climate-crisis refugees. This process continues to disenfranchise and separate Indigenous people from their ancestral lands and the traditional ecological knowledge systems they produced.

After the Treaty of Waitangi was signed in 1840, Aotearoa New Zealand was supposed to be in an equal partnership with the British Crown. Instead, the government confiscated and bought Māori land at cut-rate prices. After World War II, many young Māori moved to urban areas where they were detached from their connections to whenua through their whānau, iwi, and hapū. This injustice highlighted economic disparities between Māori and Pākehā, produced an awareness of the destructive effects of colonization, and Māori protested for restitution. In 1975, the Waitangi Tribunal was created to adjudicate cases brought by Māori individuals, iwi, or hapū, and to hear their grievances against the British Crown and the New Zealand government that had acted on its behalf since the treaty's signature in 1840. This long juridical process resulted in a series of settlements for seventy-nine claims as of December 31, 2019 (Te Tai 2020). The settlements include an acknowledgment by the Crown and the iwi in question that "full compensation for grievances is not possible. Instead, financial redress focuses on providing an economic base for iwi for future development" (Latest Treaty Settlement Bill 2019). The redress claims include a variety of options for redress through the form of grants to the iwi, including marae, education, grants to *kaumātua* (respected tribal elders), and community and cultural grants. For the purposes of this book, I focus on the marae.

While the most basic translation of *marae* is simply a meeting ground, a marae encompasses much more than that. Marae are the focal point of many Māori communities throughout Aotearoa New Zealand. Indeed, Māori people see their marae as *tūrangawaewae*—their place to stand and belong, a foundational place where Māori feel especially empowered and connected (Te Ahukaramū 2007b). Using the marae as a space for community agriculture according to Māori principles has been a way to converge culture, education, healthy food, and community in the past decade. For example, one of Tāhuri Whenua's main missions—originally called the National Māori Vegetable Growers Collective—is to "support Māori Business Development in the horticulture sector through provision of advice and information" (Roskruge 2009). The idea is to promote private-sector dissemination of information and to work within the capitalist system to ensure that Māori farmers and horticulturalists obtain their fair share of the profits in Aotearoa New Zealand as a whole. This is a vastly different perspective than Te Mahi Māra Hua Parakore, an educational program explored in greater detail in Chapter 3 that often relies on marae for educational meeting spaces. In either case, however, there can be no meaningful discussion of food production unless we are honest about the fact that the land was taken from Māori people to begin with (King 2020). Overcoming the hurdles placed by colonization and ensuring access to land, to fisheries, and to the relevant *whakapapa* (genealogies) is the first step in redressing the wrongs committed by the colonizers.

Numerous structural barriers prevent new farmers from taking on land: land-use policy is stuck in the colonial past and geared toward ownership of large tracts of land; water continues to be diverted to irrigate golf courses and for the tourist industry, or polluted by conventional livestock farming; and the state in Hawai'i and Aotearoa New Zealand are both reluctant to invest in infrastructure that would support innovative agricultural endeavors, such as food hubs or small farmer training, low-interest loans for capital improvements, or even cooperative models of equipment purchasing. We are operating in a framework stuck in an antiquated plantation mentality that is akin to the oft-quoted "get big or get out" view of agriculture. Although the politics of colonial land ownership were originally

similar in Hawai'i and Aotearoa New Zealand, current Hawai'i land-use policy
seems to be repeating the errors of the recent plantation past. Even though most
of the sugarcane plantations closed by the mid-1990s, the current decision-
makers remain focused on the status quo—supporting policies that privilege large
landowners, reproducing economies of scale using cheap labor, and avoiding any
policies that might support different models of sustainable agriculture. Instead,
policy makers should focus on understanding the plantations' failures and creating systemic conditions that will lead to sustainable agriculture for Hawai'i's
people. In Aotearoa New Zealand, Mules argues that "a lot of our postcolonial
revitalization and development has been politically inclined and quite savvy.
We're focused on governance, focused on trusts and all of these structures in the
sociopolitical space" (Mules 2020). This focus on Māori self-governance shows
how divergent the systemic solutions are in Hawai'i and Aotearoa New Zealand.
Whereas there are structures in place for iwi self-determination and sovereignty
in Aotearoa New Zealand, those political structures are only nascent in Hawai'i.
And although the Hawaiian renaissance of the late 1970s did constitutionally
mandate an Office of Hawaiian Affairs and renewed interest in Native Hawaiian
sovereignty and self-determination, the success of the semi-autonomous government office has been mixed. Mules highlights the difference:

> I think that's the difference between here and Hawai'i, which is why there isn't that
> kind of platform, so people get on with it and find a space at a real, local ground
> up level to have political assertion and it's changed our culture. You know, it's a
> different set of principles around what we value and what we think is appropriate
> for what we need in terms of culture. But causation [includes] identity and land
> and they are both just as appropriate (Mules 2020).

In both cases, then, land and identity are linked with grassroots activism that
focuses on sovereignty and self-determination. The difference in structural and
systemic barriers in each space requires different responses.

   Most of the interviewees in Hawai'i did not explicitly mention its colonial legacy,
whereas those in Aotearoa New Zealand did. Why is the narrative of colonialism
missing from the Hawai'i interview data? We could look to the sheer pervasiveness
of colonialism in Hawai'i, where street names and freeway exits are seemingly
unproblematically named for US military bases, or to Hawai'i's dependence
on imports for almost everything—not just food, but almost all manufactured
goods, fossil fuels, and tourists who supposedly "drive the economy." Perhaps

colonialism's pervasiveness in Hawai'i is what makes it invisible, whereas the critique of colonial violence in Aotearoa New Zealand is more forthright because Māori have fought for and won legal recourse for their self-determination.

Hawai'i's colonial past was nevertheless an evident undercurrent in many of the stories. For example, Monica Esquivel, a member of the Good Food Alliance in Hawai'i, and a dietetics professor at the University of Hawai'i at Mānoa, explained that she finally understood that shipping food from outside of the state meant that wealthy people and big corporate players stood to benefit from the status quo, and they would try to stop any attempts by island residents to gain self-sufficiency. She placed the struggle to change Hawai'i's food system within a capitalist economy rooted in colonialism, and essentially explained the neocolonial project as it applies to both the provenance of food and to Hawai'i's food sovereignty (Esquivel 2019).

Although neocolonialism serves as a constant reminder that the colonial history of both Hawai'i and Aotearoa New Zealand is still shaping our respective food systems, focusing on justice-oriented frameworks for food system solutions was apparent in many of the interview narratives. Several respondents echoed critiques of injustices based on economic conditions, lack of access to land ownership, poverty, and powerlessness. Alicia Higa, director of Health Promotion at the Wai'anae Coast Comprehensive Health Center, shared that the farmers' markets she promoted are not just about increasing access to food; they are "food justice markets" (Higa 2019). Indeed, Kaui Sana, the farm manager at MA'O Organic Farms on the Leeward Coast of O'ahu explained that some nonprofit organizations working in this sector are inherently based on "social justice-oriented values, environmental justice-oriented values…at this nexus point within community, here's an organization [MA'O Farms] that is intentionally manifesting on all of those levels" (Sana 2019). Even prior to doing nonprofit work in this sector, Ashley Lukens, formerly of the Hawai'i Center for Food Safety and now an independent philanthropic and development advisor, based her dissertation on food justice movements, specifically looking at work to dismantle racism and understanding her own privilege (Lukens 2019). Here, we see the relationship between privilege and allyship as an additional layer to the critique of social, political, and economic injustices around food. As Lukens (2019) explained in her interview, "for communities that might have been historically disenfranchised or, in Hawai'i, completely reject the legitimacy of the state," can allies be part of the conversation in productive and meaningful ways to foster food system trans-formation so that access to good, clean, fair food is available to all communities?

Can these conversations about voice and empowerment translate to actionable items, not just "slacktivism"? That is, when we know there is a problem, can we do more than raise awareness of it and work for change on a policy or legislative scale, or through business, or even through community activism? As Audre Lorde (1984) said, "the master's tools will never dismantle the master's house." Is it possible that completely *dismantling* the current food system in place is the only possible way forward? If there is anything to learn from the women interviewed for this project, it is precisely that women in Oceania are taking matters into their own hands and finding creative ways of engaging each other, as well as their respective communities, to make changes; find solutions to the problems created by colonialism, capitalism, racism, discrimination; and center food as a source of both nourishment and a powerful force for transformation and justice.

Respondents in Aotearoa New Zealand were explicit in their discussion of colonialism's legacy. Dr. Matire Harwood, a general practitioner at Papakura Marae Health Clinic in South Auckland and an Associate Professor of Medicine at the University of Auckland, explained that

> if you look back in time, there was a part of colonization that wiped out the legal abilities of people to look after themselves. A lot of the gardens were torched to try and prevent it from happening. The wonderful farmland was stolen and given to the war veterans as they came back but not to Māori, who also participated in the war. (Harwood 2020)

This legally sanctioned dispossession of land led to a series of additional problems within marginalized Māori communities. Most importantly, however, the loss of land broke the family connection between the whenua and Māori people. Kelly Francis is the director of an organization called Whenua Warrior that organizes and builds gardens around Auckland. I interviewed her shortly after my arrival in Auckland, at Ihumātao Village, a space that resists Māori land dispossession by occupying the area where the developer Fletcher Building seized Crown lands (Latif 2020). Francis shared that her work at Ihumātao Village taught her that there are injustices everywhere and that she can use this knowledge to help people. She also said there should never have been a Māori word to translate "land ownership" because the concept runs counter to Māori values. This colonial history was front and center when Hineāmaru Ropati (2020), a Hua Parakore teacher at Mangere East Papatūānuku Kōkiri Marae, explained how and why the land was lost:

They saw the Māori growing food as a major threat because it was making an impact on their trading. It's all about money and capital as it is. And it made a big impact on our food, so we lost a lot of our lands. And over time we lost a lot of our lives. We lost the lore about planting. On top of that, we lost those links because they're mass planting like monoculture and not inter-species planting at all like we did in the past. (Ropati 2020)

Beyond the dispossession of land, colonial violence in Aotearoa New Zealand applies global capitalist values to the food system. Angela Clifford, the executive director of Eat New Zealand, a nonprofit food movement dedicated to connecting people to Aotearoa New Zealand through food, explained it as follows:

The Ministry of Food did a deal with the Marketing Department of New Zealand and that pretty much encapsulates absolutely everything about how we see ourselves as a food nation. We're a trading economy, always have been. But we lack our own self-identity because we are pretty much the paddock and an ocean for the "motherland." It's just that the motherland changed over the years. We had this unfortunate relationship with ourselves in terms of how we see ourselves. We just lack our own self-identity and that plays out constantly. It means that we end up exporting a list of ingredients and not talking about who we are and what we were originally. A lot of our stories and people and ingredients have been buried. And we really have no idea how rich and diverse that was. We sort of covered it over with a very colonized version of our food story, which revolves around pastures and stuff for the motherland. (Clifford 2020)

Clifford's reflection on the colonial food story highlights that there is not only a significant loss of land, but a loss of stories and knowledge that erases Indigenous foodways and traditions and replaces them with a sanitized version of exported foods for the "motherland" grown on the green pastures typically associated with the lore of Aotearoa New Zealand. Whether those pastures are polluted by overgrazing or high-intensity livestock or dairy production does not factor into the image of Aotearoa New Zealand's food stories, even though they are very much a part of the reality.

The colonized version of our food story is that we've lost our Indigenous and our original stories, for all intents and purposes and those Indigenous stories that remain have become quiet. They're the shell of themselves in terms of stories. There's two or three that are left, but it in no way reflects the diversity and richness. (Clifford 2020)

Clifford's job is to highlight the diversity of food stories in Aotearoa New Zealand and to make them connect with worldwide audiences. She laments the loss of the stories, which threatens the loss of the culture itself.

Hawai'i and Aotearoa New Zealand Food System Snapshots

Much is often made of the fact that Hawai'i imports anywhere between 85% and 90% of its food. Under former Governor Ige's 2016 mandate, the state plans to double local food production by 2030 (Terrell 2021), but statistics show that local food production has declined significantly, from 175,207,000 pounds at the beginning of 1996 (when records started being kept), to 67,205,000 pounds produced at the end of 2018, with an all-time high of over 200,000,000 pounds in 1998 (Local Foods Production Dashboard 2025). Doubling food production from current production levels of 10% would not even approximate 1996 levels. Additionally, there is a high degree of variability in the kinds of foods Hawai'i produces locally. Whereas the local seafood industry provides 55% of Hawai'i's fish consumption, the local meat and dairy industries provide only a very small percentage of current meat and milk consumption. Fruits and vegetables account for a larger share of locally consumed foods, but are still well below acceptable rates. Hawai'i does produce specialty crops, though many of those (coffee, maca-damia nuts, pineapples, papayas) are for export. These dire statistics indicate that something must be done—and soon—to reverse these trends, because Hawai'i is particularly vulnerable to climate change and natural disasters, along with fuel price fluctuations and other potential economic and shipping disruptions.

With an abundance of food being grown in Aotearoa New Zealand, why con-ceptualize as problematic something that is so pervasive and available in people's lives? Indeed, the country's political establishment pushes the idea that food is "plentiful, apolitical, local, and environmentally sound" (Bartos 2016, 93). Emily King explained to me that Aotearoa New Zealand residents have yet to realize the importance of food systems. However, much of the literature on Aotearoa New Zealand's food system acknowledges similar problems to those found in Hawai'i. Much of this literature tends to focus on the ever-present deficit model: food insecurity leads to high rates of nutrition-related chronic diseases in Māori communities (Stevenson 2011; Glover et al. 2019; Vandevijvere et al. 2019); the lack of culturally appropriate foods available exacerbates these problems (Bartos 2016; Healthy Families NZ 2023); conventional agriculture is environmentally

(Hutchings 2015) and nutritionally (Jones et al. 2019) unsustainable. Māori food sovereignty offers a promising contrast to this work. Focusing on the positive attributes of a more sustainable, just, and healthy Māori food system has the potential to revitalize sustainable agriculture for *all* of Aotearoa New Zealand's people (Bartos 2016; Huambachano 2018, 2019; Lyver et al. 2017; Moeke-Pickering et al. 2015; Shirley 2013).

Mules emphasizes that focusing on AFNs is the way forward:

> Mostly in that kind of gardening space, because it was traditionally a subsistence economy with big staple "feed the masses" type gardening. We've got the *kūmara* (sweet potato). A little bit of taro with big populations, strong boundary lines, all of the stuff that comes with horticultural societies. In 2013, [when she did her MA thesis research] there was still some of the old farmers around here who had seen those gardens, who had worked in the big gardens and still pined for them. Everyone I interviewed now has passed on, and with them, we lost a lot of those lived experiences. I really looked at how you can use environmental advancement and how it can be a marker for the health of the community. Gardening can be a tool to measure well-being and help how people use the land and on what scale. My community still desires and has a cultural foundation and true deep-seated passion for working the land. (Mules 2020)

Māori gardening traditions, which foster a sustainable horticultural society through Indigenous ecological knowledge, are still there, but they are waning. Many of the respondents—and especially Mules, who did graduate work on Māori horticultural systems—saw that this was a moment rife for intervention, whether through formal Māori governance, community input, or a combination of both. Losing the lived experience of Māori gardeners is akin to losing the ancestral knowledge necessary to reclaim food sovereignty.

> If you were to go through some kind of revitalization of the local community, food systems would be your platform. It's a given because food comes from the land. These two are so intertwined. All of those things are the low hanging fruit. You can't deny that food is intertwined with culture. And culture is also intertwined with tradition and tradition is often stuck in time…Our culture knows gardening is something so much more complex. If you could tap into that, people are gonna turn up and work. They're gonna turn up and feed the elderly. They're going to turn up and do the hard yards. (Mules 2020)

Mules's discussion of the connection between gardening culture and Māori foodways is critical because it highlights how that connection has the potential to transform food systems. She argues that relying on Indigenous knowledge about sustainable agriculture and food production enables people to connect the land to their family genealogy. This engages Māori with their traditions and fosters participation in sustainable community food systems to benefit iwi, hapū, and whānau.

Some argue for policy change at various levels of government—that is, top-down style interventions combined with grassroots and community interventions from the bottom up to create and maintain meaningful changes to the food system (Stevenson 2011). Certainly, this is the case for most large-scale systemic changes. One cannot create change in a vacuum or without support from various entities, starting from the individual, moving to community, and then to private and public sector levels. Furthermore, Shirley (2013) argues that "inherent in a food system is culture, language and identity" (60). That encompasses just about everything relevant to people's daily lives, no matter where they live, but it is especially important in a neocolonial context where Indigenous peoples have been marginalized. To ensure a response based on culturally appropriate knowledge systems, Hutchings (2015) asserts six pillars of Māori food sovereignty: the focus should be on food for the people, not for export; the value of food providers should be emphasized; local food systems are key to bringing consumers and producers together; there should be local control over ways to produce sustainable agricultural products and maintain diversity; local food producers need support to build their knowledge and skills for managing local food production; and everyone should work with nature to improve resilience and adaptation. These building blocks are rooted in Māori culture and present in Kanaka Maoli culture as well. Creation stories or cosmologies explain why and how these systems are to be maintained and fostered in the face of a global capitalist system that devalues smallholder production and instead encourages larger and larger farms that mostly grow food for export.

Women in the Food System

Women work as garden educators in schools, organic farmers, teachers, lawyers fighting for food justice, policy makers, cafeteria managers, food hub managers, compost builders, grant writers in the food and agriculture space, seed savers, farmers' market managers and vendors, and a host of other food system related occupations. This work pushes Hawai'i and Aotearoa New Zealand toward a more just and sustainable food future focused on food sovereignty. Learning from Indigenous agricultural practices also encourages us to look at the roles of women in Kanaka Maoli and Māori cultures in order to understand how to transform the food systems in these two island ecosystems. As Lilikalā Kame'eleihiwa writes in *Nā Wāhine Kapu: Divine Hawaiian Women*, "[a]s Hawaiian women, we are the intellectual as well as the physical descendants of our female ancestors, and in turn we will be ancestral inspiration for the generations to come. This is the Hawaiian and Polynesian way, and it is the heart of our cultural identity" (1999, 1). This view places value on the work and words of Kanaka Maoli women in determining the future. In their emphasis on the connection between land and nourishment in Hawai'i, women's narratives are particularly salient to debates surrounding the future of Hawai'i's food system. As in Mules's narrative about the power of women's roles in Māori cosmology, Native Hawaiian genealogy and history highlights the importance of the relationship between land, humans, and food. For example, Kame'eleihiwa explains that

> Papahānaumoku: Papa the woman who gives birth to islands, Papa the earth mother who mates with her brother Wākea, the sky father and to whom are born the Hawaiian Islands, the sacred *kalo* plant, and the Hawaiian people. It is Papahānaumoku who agrees to Wākea's suggestion of the new religion called *'Aikapu*, and to the separation of male and female in labor, in cooking, in food, and in sacrifice. The *'Aikapu*, or sacred eating, makes the eating of food a religious experience, a communion with the gods, surrounded by ceremony and constraint. (1999, 7, emphasis in original)

The act of eating food is a sacred experience; we need food to sustain our bodies and our spiritual selves. The Kanaka Maoli cosmology excerpt, taken together with the stories of Kanaka Maoli and Māori women as well as the diverse women working in this field, are critical to understanding the landscape of Hawai'i's and Aotearoa New Zealand's AFNs.

Women have always been a part of Oceania's agricultural reality, but they have remained unseen and unheard. *Feeding Hawai'i* published a blog post by Pomai Weigert, an Ag Business consultant with GoFarm Hawai'i, whom *Forbes* magazine named as one of the five female leaders of Hawai'i's agriculture scene. Weigert writes that women are the "unsung heroes and boss ladies in this business and they are no longer 'behind the scenes.' They bring a different energy, vision and vitality to an industry that has been male-dominated for generations" (2025). This is not to say that the agricultural industry itself has been exclusively male-dominated; women have participated in it in meaningful ways, from before European contact to the present day, but, there is a dearth of academic literature on women, food systems, and agriculture in Hawai'i. For example, a library database search of the key words "women," "gender," "agriculture," "Hawai'i," "food system," or any combination thereof produces less than ten results, six of which are medical journal articles concerning the fertility of certain microbes, or the male fertility of invasive insects in the tropics. Clearly, there is a gap in the literature that needs to be filled with the work and stories of women in the food system in Oceania.

Prior to European contact, Kanaka Maoli women were integral parts of an intricately connected system of land stewardship—the '*aikapu* (forbidden, sacred, or holy) system—in which growing and distributing food provided abundant resources to almost a million people. Without their work, the system would not have been able to thrive as it did, with each person knowing and understanding their roles within a loop of plenty. Native Hawaiian cosmology asserts that

> the Hawaiian world was thereafter divided into female and male domains of work, and was considered *pono*, correct and righteous, when there was a balance between the two. When there is balance in the world, the ancestral *Akua* [gods, spirits] are pleased, and when there is perfect harmony in the universe, people are protected from all harm. (Kame'eleihiwa 1999, 4)

Recreating that balance between land and people is critical to overhauling Hawai'i's food system. Rooting this balance in the tradition of ancestral abundance, especially through the use of the *ahupua'a* (traditionally, a wedge-shaped portion of land that included mountainous regions with watersheds, low-lying irrigated areas near shore for agricultural systems, and ocean access for fishing) system is also key to transitioning to a sustainable food system that feeds Hawai'i's people with healthy and just foods.

Upon their arrival, American missionaries insisted on forcibly changing Kanaka Maoli women's roles to align with their own western sensibilities. Women were no longer allowed to surf naked alongside their male counterparts. Hula, an artistic expression of stories and culture, was banned, as was speaking or teaching the Hawaiian language in schools. When I first started teaching at the University of Hawai'i at Mānoa in 1997, a student told me that she was forbidden from speaking 'Ōlelo Hawai'i in her home by her grandmother, who had been beaten for doing so during her own childhood. She did not want her children and grandchildren to suffer the same fate. This particular student took it upon herself to learn 'Ōlelo Hawai'i at Kamehameha Schools, unbeknownst to her family, who insisted she take Japanese because it was considered the language of "success" at the time. Because language is a critical component of cultural renaissance, this student's act of resistance against her family was a way for her to maintain her relationship with the Hawaiian culture and ensure its survival, at least within her family.

This story is all too familiar in Hawai'i, although thankfully attitudes toward Hawaiian-ness have become much more positive, due in part to the Hawaiian cultural renaissance of the late 1970s, the centennial protests against the illegal overthrow of the Hawaiian monarchy in 1993, and unlawful annexation by the US in 1998. The impact of the missionaries and their policies to force Hawaiian women into the "cult of true womanhood" to fit their ideas of femininity are still evident, however, given the erasure of women's lives and contributions to the food system in Hawai'i (Grimshaw 1989). To remedy these glaring omissions, a small yet significant number of scholars are working to amplify Native stories. For example, University of Hawai'i Political Science professor Noenoe Silva rediscovered the Kū'ē Petitions against annexation hidden in the National Archives in 1998. They included about 95% of the Native adult population of Hawai'i at the time, which overwhelmingly opposed annexation. This indicates that there is a long, often ignored history of resistance to colonization in Hawai'i (Silva 2004). The petitions included both men's and women's signatures protesting the annexation of the Kingdom of Hawai'i to the US. Missionaries' earlier demands for "propriety" had not subdued women. Their strength in resistance has remained steadfast in the face of oppression by the various forces coming to Hawai'i. This work is ongoing and inhabits many different practices.

Women can support and uplift each other in the food system space in various ways. For example, Frankie Koethe at the O'ahu Resources Defense Council explains that her organization set up the Hawai'i Women Farmers' Workshop Series and its related Facebook group so that women can rely on each other as resources for a variety of agricultural experiences.

> About three years ago, we started to see a switch in the statistics of women in agriculture in Hawai'i through the US Census, and we were starting to see an increase in numbers, and we thought that it may be something we should look at a little bit closer. We did an initial survey of the risk management concerns for women in agriculture and had about one hundred twenty-five respondents from around the state. (Koethe 2019)

Using data-driven decision-making to surmise that women were starting to become farmers in greater numbers, the Oʻahu Resources Defense Council started a program to cater to their specific needs, finding out what kinds of issues they were interested in, and what kinds of resources they might need.

> We set up the Women Farmers' Workshop and we basically did a tour of farms for monthly workshops and brought presenters with us that could speak on those topics. It was really good for new, beginning farmers, or people who needed to brush up on these topics, but we found the most powerful thing that came from it was the talking. (Koethe 2019)

Community-driven input from the different farmers in their networks engaged all of the participants in a process of teaching and learning that enabled farmers to help each other, share stories and experiences, and explain the challenges and opportunities they faced.

> We used that to spearhead our women farmers' network. We created the Facebook group that has about 180 members right now, mostly farmers, and some women like farmer advocates and professionals who need resources. The goal is that they keep these conversations going and bring more women so that they can lean on each other and really be a resource. (Koethe 2019)

The networking and connection aspects of these groups ensure that knowledge is passed on from farmer to farmer on all islands. This may include applying certain sustainable agricultural practices, sharing information about grant-funding opportunities, or simply having someone to talk to who might be facing similar pest or plant disease issues.

Many respondents spoke about relying on their respective support networks to increase their respective capacities for success. Indeed, Tina Tamai, the director of the Good Food Alliance calls her group

> a network of networks. Everybody wants to be engaged in good food and provide good access and promote healthy eating because we have really strong people in our network. The intent is to try to do a shared leadership model. (Tamai 2019)

According to Tamai, the network of networks idea stems from two related issues. The first is that if the Good Food Alliance were to include everyone interested in improving Hawaiʻi's food system, there would simply be too many people at the meetings, and nothing would get accomplished. Second, each of the representatives from the participating organizations have known each other for a long time and have worked well together since the inception of the Good Food Alliance.

> It's that thing about women nurturing and the connection of philosophy based on food is important because I think most of the people in our group are foodies. They value food and they value good food for their children. I think that's how you get started. I want my kids to eat healthy food. I want my grandkids to eat healthy, too. What we're doing is we're trying to support food systems to create better access and to promote healthy eating in low-income communities to create better access to healthy food. (Tamai 2019)

Like Cole and others who mentioned women's nurturing, Tamai explains that this is a source of strength, rather than a liability.

> I think that's at the heart of things, and I think women are very strong. I think that a lot of the women, because they're kind of detailed and at the same time have a goal, they can make the connections better. At least for the women, what we have in common in our lives is that all those skill sets, both sets: the detail and the systems-thinking. And being able to be sensitive to people's feelings and what their needs are because the whole idea of building a food system is that you have to see what the gaps are and be sensitive to what people are wanting and need, and to piece that together to make a system that works that meets people's goals and needs. But our question is how do we sustain it? (Tamai 2019)

That last question in Tamai's narrative is likely the most important aspect of this research project. Without continuous grant funding, how do these projects remain afloat? How does the value of a healthy food system drive itself to be both sustainable and profitable so that people can afford to be both producers *and* consumers of local food? As Meleana Judd, owner of Waihuena Farm on the North Shore of Oʻahu, says, "the place is as much of a product as the produce" (Judd 2019). (Re)creating a foodscape with Indigenous values at the center and fostering an appreciation for Hawaiʻi's agricultural products while ensuring they are affordable and accessible to all is clearly difficult to accomplish. Nevertheless, Hawaiʻi's leaders in the food system change movement (many of whom are women) are working together to foster those changes and continuing to learn from each other.

Highlighting this link between land and women does not necessarily throw us back to an earlier time where that relationship might have been seen as a deficit. Nor does it push us toward essentialist ecofeminist principles. Instead, as Johnston and Pihama (2019) so rightly argue:

> As Māori women we each have a relationship to the land; we are each connected to mana whenua. As Māori women we have a relationship to spirituality, mana wairua. As Māori women we are located in complex relationships within whaka-papa, mana tangata. Each of these aspects of tikanga Māori is a part of who we are as Māori women, whether or not we experience them in our day-to-day real-ities, as they originate from historical and cultural sources that both precede and succeed us. The complexities of such relationships extend into whānau, hapū and iwi, so no single expression is the "one"; all of them may, and do, find a range of expressions. Hence, what may be viewed as an essence in cultural terms does not, in our terms, equate to essentialism. Rather, it expresses the historical and social construction of cultural relationships (Johnston and Pihama 2019, 165)

An Indigenous feminist perspective turns (mostly white) western feminist per-spectives, with their deficit models associated with Mother Earth essentialism, on their heads. Kate Cherrington explained that "[i]t's just a Māori way of thinking and being with the land and growing food. So we are in a relationship that was absolutely genealogically based on family connection, which is really important and grows naturally" (Cherrington 2020). Mules's postcolonial feminist Māori creation story interpretation, Cherrington's direct explanation of the epistemo-logical underpinnings of the family connection between land and people, and Johnston and Pihama's view of how family is relevant and applied to women's lives, combine to tell a formidable story about women's roles in food system reform efforts throughout Oceania.

The interviewees from Aotearoa New Zealand identified many of the sustainable agricultural innovations as being spearheaded by women. Trish Allen, co-founder of Rainbow Valley Farm, a large organic farm using regenerative agricultural practices on the North Island, sold the farm after her partner passed away and moved to a small town a short distance away. But given her long history with sustainable agriculture, she ended up starting a community garden in the town just a few years later.

> One of the things that I did when I left Rainbow Valley Farm and moved to the village, together with a woman friend, was to start a community garden here in

the village. We started it back in 2012. And actually, it's mostly women who come
along to that garden every week. It's not a huge garden. It's quite small, and we
garden together. And we grow vegetables and fruit, and we share it all out. We
meet once a week on a Monday morning. And it's only an hour and a half or
two hours. But we have such a lovely time, and we share ideas. And that is all
women. Occasionally we'll get a man come along. Not very often, but mostly
it's women. (Allen 2020)

Similarly, Jessica Barnes, the community/market garden manager at For The
Better Good, in Wellington, asserts that women are locked out of other public
spaces, so they turn to gardens and community in order to nourish their families
and their communities.

I think that kind of is a reflection as a caregiver and that extends to caregiver
of the entire earth, which includes a lot of emotional labor. I do wonder on a
larger scale that women are sometimes more innovative because they're locked
out of other spaces on government policy levels. I don't know what the ratio of
women are in those spaces, but it does feel more male-centered perhaps than
female-centered. (Barnes 2020)

Jenny Lux, the co-owner of Lux Organics, an organic farm in Rotorua, asserted
that the unbroken tradition of women passing down gardening and agricultural
knowledge runs deep in both Māori and Pākehā communities.

I became interested in gardening when I was a child with my mother. We always
kept the connection to the land. I come from an unbroken line of Irish immigrant
farming, gardening families. My grandmother grew food for the family and passed
on the knowledge about how to grow food for the family to my mom. My mom
did that for me. There's been no break in that whole chain. (Lux 2020)

This generational thinking epitomizes an anti-capitalist, anti-colonial perspective,
yet it is deployed as a strategy for understanding her place in life as an organic
farmer and a white settler to Aotearoa New Zealand. Although conflicts over
land ownership remain, the connection between land and family is central to all
of these narratives, no matter whether the impetus starts from Māori or Pākehā
cultural traditions.

Conclusion

The language of co-production in sustainable community food systems under-scores that producers need consumers and, of course, consumers need producers. The equation at the root of this basic economic model shows the importance of each one's dependency on the other for survival, not in a way that is exploited for profit. Valuing connectedness through food systems means recognizing that we exist in a relationship with others and with the land. This mindset is not new to Indigenous peoples all over the world or throughout Oceania. Yet through the narratives, a different picture emerges of respondents' views of that relationship.

In Hawai'i, the narrative surrounding colonization and its impact on food systems is present, but the respondents do not explicitly mention it. Partly, this is due to the sheer pervasiveness of the American colonization experience—it is so present in everyday life that we no longer see its active and ongoing processes. In Aotearoa New Zealand, many of the narratives highlight the injustices of British colonialism—namely, that it led to Māori land dispossession. Centering the process of colonization means that it can also be *de*centered in our discourse, and we can actively resist against it. This has the potential to serve food system reform efforts, because if we can see something happening, we can actually do something to change it.

CHAPTER 2

Land Stewardship: Mālama 'Āina and Kaitiakitanga Whenua

*E mālama 'oe I ka 'Āina, e Mālama ka 'Āina ia 'oe / Take care of the land and the
land will take care of you.*
—'Ōlelo No'eau/Hawaiian proverb

Nourishing the Soil, Nourishing the People

Throughout the research process for this book, the concept of nourishment emerged as a primary focus for many of the interviewees. They interpreted nourishment differently: in terms of feeding families or feeding people on a larger scale, such as school food programs, and in terms of nourishing the soil, either in practical terms through composting programs or regenerative agriculture to improve soil and crop quality, or in more spiritual terms like nourishing the land by paying attention to its needs and performing culturally appropriate chants or *oli* (spoken word chant) prior to starting work on a farm. Ku'ulei Samson, a program manager and garden education teacher at Hoa 'Āina O Mākaha, a five-acre organic school garden adjacent to Mākaha Elementary school on the Leeward Coast of O'ahu, shared that nourishing the soil and people are "really just cycles, cycles of life. The plants reflect so much that once we come into the garden, now we're able to bear a relationship with the soil" (Samson 2020). Through this process, Samson tells visitors to the farm that they will end up creating community because once they start growing food, they will realize that they cannot eat it all and will end up sharing it with their neighbors and community, making friends in the process. She equates this to the

> Hawaiian culture when we had these ranks of different people, and those people were meant to have those different responsibilities…[and] just that act of being able to bring people up to your level so that you're able to step into higher responsibilities so that they can step up higher with you. (Samson 2020)

Supporting and uplifting community through ʻāina work fosters and nourishes lasting relationships. It also nurtures leaders within communities who promote sustainable agriculture and other AFNs. For instance, Dana Shapiro, the ʻUlu Cooperative director on Hawaiʻi Island, stated that women are

> Thinking about food and nourishing and feeding their own families. And I think naturally that extends more broadly to the food system. I think women oftentimes focus their energy on really practical needs and material needs. As they look around at all the needs and the problems and the challenges facing our society, food is a super concrete and basic fact of life. It doesn't necessarily require super high-tech solutions. And women are kind of like nuts and bolts. It often involves a lot of just community organizing and "people work." How do we get people to come together around a shared problem and shared goals and work together? I do think that women are better at bringing people together. Then also, the solutions that women see and maybe prioritize are the ones that are more community-oriented than technology-augmented. (Shapiro 2019)

Shapiro uses strategic essentialism to tie together the gendered aspects of collaborative work to accomplish the goal of transforming the food system. Following the idea of intersectional praxis, if the work is getting done, that is what matters to her, not necessarily who is doing it. It just so happens that the people doing the food system transformation work, in Shapiro's view, are mostly women.

> I think our contribution is really more about the collaboration that has emerged and that is being cultivated through the projects. And oftentimes, I think women are more collaborative. Men tend to see things more through a competition lens. Women are like, how can we just work together to get this done right? (Shapiro 2019)

Shapiro believes that nourishment stems from collaboration, and that the food system is a concrete space where women can implement creative solutions that will produce positive changes. She establishes a counternarrative of value and worth in collaboration, instead of focusing on competition and profits, arguing that this is how the work gets done. Collaborating with women in other food system spaces means that they are nourishing people by providing access to healthy and culturally appropriate local food. This example emphasizes the political project of intersectional FPE praxis. The women work together to accomplish their goals, and to ensure food system change, whether in small regional ways, or through larger, statewide means.

'Ulu, or breadfruit (*Artocarpus altilis*), is a starchy, tropical tree fruit, ranging from the size of a softball to the size of a small basketball depending on the variety, with green skin and a cream-colored interior. It can be eaten at any stage of its development in either savory or sweet preparations. When roasted, it smells like freshly baked bread, hence the name. It was a staple crop for Hawaiians until the 1950s and remains an important food source throughout the rest of Oceania to this day. Interest in its nutritional and sustainability benefits have undergone a resurgence in Hawai'i during the last few decades. It is now being substituted for imported potatoes in some school lunch dishes, thereby fostering a large institutional demand for the crop. Diane Ragone of the Breadfruit Institute, at both Maui and Kaua'i's National Tropical Botanical Garden research stations, has worked tirelessly since 2003 to promote 'ulu as a culturally appropriate crop for Pacific peoples that can help alleviate hunger on a global scale, as well as "support regenerative agriculture, food security, and economic development in the tropics" (National Tropical Botanical Garden 2020). 'Ulu is a central component of traditional agroforestry throughout Oceania. Indeed, there are approximately 150 varieties in existence, all with their own cultural cooking and preparation traditions. 'Ulu trees are pest and disease resistant, and with little upkeep can provide food to a community for fifty years, with no annual replanting. Ragone's work led to a resurgence of 'ulu as an in-demand crop and Shapiro's work at the 'Ulu Cooperative capitalized on this trend. This crop is essential to nourishing people and reinvigorating culture through connection with ancestral foodways.

Shapiro explains her role and the structure of the 'Ulu Cooperative this way:

> I manage a farmer co-op. We have about eighty-five farmer members, mostly on the Big Island, a couple on Maui. And we just made our three-year anniversary [in 2019]. We're still a really young organization, but we basically aggregate our farmers' 'ulu and we process it to extend the season and shelf life and add some value. Mostly we just do minimal processing, steaming, and freezing and then we distribute. We do all the public schools in the state, a bunch of private schools, hospitals and then various restaurants and hotels and we're really just getting into retail sales. We do freezer pouches for grocery stores that we're just launching now. (Shapiro 2019)

'Ulu is quite prevalent in less westernized and less occupied spaces in Oceania, though it has been lost as a staple crop in Hawai'i and replaced with white rice. To remedy this situation, the 'Ulu Cooperative does "a ton of education. 'Ulu is not really a staple crop for [the] whole school system anymore. Most people don't know how to prepare it or even don't know about it, or maybe have like a negative connotation" (Shapiro 2019). Shapiro examined co-op model structures for her master's degree. She was able to apply that knowledge to the Hawai'i food system to create a space where small producers could come together to make use of facilities using economies of scale, instead of having to purchase expensive equipment individually.

> To me, the co-op business model is really, really well-suited to the food system. Because in Hawai'i, 96 percent of our farmers are super small scale. And co-ops make sense when you have a large quantity of small-scale producers, consumers, buyers, who basically band together to increase their collective bargaining power and so forth. For the food system as a whole, I think co-ops really are key to improvement in that sphere. (Shapiro 2019)

The cooperative takes care of education, marketing, distributing, and sales, for a cut of the profits. When Shapiro and I talked story, the cooperative had seventeen employees and was looking to expand to another warehouse on the other side of Hawai'i Island, where it would presumably hire additional employees. The co-op is itself a site of resistance to the industrial agro-food system since its premise rests on bringing back production and consumption of a traditional Native Hawaiian crop. As Shapiro explains, " 'Ulu is not a new crop. Obviously, it's an ancient crop. But it's been lost. You know, so inserting a new crop into food that is already served in schools and or reheated in schools, I feel like it's pushing against the current food system" (Shapiro 2019). Simply by virtue of using 'ulu as a staple instead of as a specialty food, the cooperative is doing its part to decolonize Hawai'i's food system, as well as ensuring income for small 'ulu producers who sell to the cooperative, educating children in schools about its role as a staple crop in ancient Hawaiian foodways, and feeding people good, local food by making it easy to cook. 'Ulu can be somewhat hard to manage in the kitchen. It's a bit messy, with a sticky sap if the 'ulu is even slightly unripe, yet not only is it delicious, but it can be eaten in a myriad of ways, and at all different times in its lifecycle. The cooperative's focus on pre-quartered or pre-cut frozen 'ulu pieces make it more accessible to people who don't have an 'ulu tree in their yard, as well as to institutional buyers like school cafeterias, prisons, and hospitals where it can easily be substituted for imported potatoes. The "winners" here are both the producers who have an outlet for their 'ulu crops, and the consumers, who get to eat a delicious, locally grown, and culturally appropriate food.

Without nourishing the soil, growing food is impossible. In some spaces, the soil needed to pursue sustainable agriculture was already in good condition; for example, Hannah Zwartz, the Urban Kai Garden coordinator in Lower Hutt, near Wellington in Aotearoa New Zealand, had an advantage in creating her garden because the area had been a market garden prior to being developed with housing (Zwartz 2020). In other places, the soil needed serious remediation. Based on purely anecdotal evidence, gleaned from traveling around the North Island for almost three weeks conducting talk story sessions, there seemed to be more of a focus on composting and waste recycling in Aotearoa New Zealand than in Hawai'i. There were recycling and compost bins in public places and private homes, as well as every organization I visited. Kate Walmsley, the compost guru at Kaicycle, also in Wellington, gave a nuanced explanation of the additional benefits of nourishing the soil:

> That was really the entry point to me—the biological processes that are involved in composting which then led into how composting is improving soil health. How are ecosystem health and food security and social well-being and water quality and climate change linked? Everything is an ecosystem and it's really helped me realize how everything is connected. (Walmsley 2020)

This view addresses both the ecosystem services inherent in the composting process as well as the inclusion of humans in the food system to highlight how they are all tied together. This holistic perspective fosters a growing awareness of the importance of systems-thinking to address global problems like climate change, local problems like diverting the waste stream to compost hubs that necessarily involves humans with the ecosystem, and the well-being of specific communities, water pollution, or soil health.

> In the western capitalist model, we tend to look at things very discretely and in different packages and those are the very things that lead to soil degradation. That has been linked to so many of the problems we're currently experiencing today, like food, poverty, and waterways—soil loss and waterway pollution. (Walmsley 2020)

Walmsley connects the short-term perspective inherent in capitalism and the necessary long-term view of nourishing the soil to nourish the people. Composting and regenerative agriculture take more time than conventional agriculture, so thinking in the short-term is clearly not an option.

> And I mean, going a bit deeper, unhappiness and loneliness, obesity and all these things can be so overwhelming when you look at everything as discrete issues. But then, you realize that these changes, all these problems are interlinked. We can act on all of them by using some data on these underlying issues, one of which is soil health. How we perceive the soil is how we perceive the ecosystem around us.
>
> Soil degradation is a huge issue and there's also a massive compost deficit. I see my role and a role of a lot of us in this space in New Zealand to really champion composting. I don't want to use the word "fight against," but present composting as a much better solution in so many ways before we invest heavily into equipment which locks us into biogas production. (Walmsley 2020)

Improved soil health doesn't occur overnight, so working on nourishing the soil has long-term implications. It also involves consistent attention and tending—as Walmsley explains, because humans live within ecosystems, even urban ones, and understanding how we live in nature, and how systems are linked is critical to our future health and well-being. Interestingly, she echoes Shapiro's claim that men are looking for technological and machine-based solutions.

> The critical energy investment right now across New Zealand, is that we're seeing a lot of interest in biogas production from food waste. A lot of it is waste to energy which is not feeding that circular economy because there is no nutrient recovery.
>
> It's such an easier solution to say, "oh here is a machine that we can buy. It's gonna cost a lot but we know how to buy things and we know how to use bank loans." I think maybe women are perhaps more willing, or perhaps better at imagining, painting a broader picture and taking a lot of other factors into consideration. Maybe men are more into machines, but they're kind of groomed that way from a young age, right? In the urban context, people are generally more into machines. What you see as unappealing is behind a wall, and you just have something nice come out. Composting gets a really bad rap but that's just because it's often misunderstood and poorly done. (Walmsley 2020)

Walmsley sees her role as a "compost champion" as central to improving policy about food systems and energy production, because she is making sure policymakers understand the importance of using waste for composting and soil regeneration (instead of burning waste to create energy). This process improves soil health, leading to healthier crops and healthier people, and offers a long-term, low-cost solution to food waste, especially in urban areas. Investing large sums of money in heavy equipment for biogas production to burn waste and turn it into energy is a short-term solution to a long-term problem.

Mālama ʻāina and Kaitiakitanga Whenua

Mālama ʻāina means to care for the land in ʻŌlelo Hawaiʻi. *Kaitiakitanga whenua* focuses on guardianship and conservation of the land in Te Reo Māori. These are basic literal translations—easily accomplished with Google Translate. Both concepts exist in Hawaiʻi and Aotearoa New Zealand, with slight variations in the applications of the terms. However, their present-day uses are not the same. Mālama ʻāina has been coopted by almost every entity in Hawaiʻi in an attempt to greenwash their practices. At the same time, numerous nonprofit organizations that do serious environmental restoration work also use this terminology. They pay attention to the spiritual and traditional practices necessary to respectfully enter certain spaces, chanting oli to reflect genealogies and ask permission to enter from the existing stewards of the space. In Aotearoa New Zealand, kaitiakitanga as an act includes the "guardianship by the tangata whenua (people of the land) of an area in accordance with tikanga Māori [Māori customary practices and behaviors] in relation to natural and physical resources; and includes the ethic of stewardship" (Te Ahukaramū 2007a). Pākehā settlers may have different worldviews on natural resource management, and land stewardship has not been coopted as aggressively by greenwashing corporations as it has in Hawaiʻi.

The tension between genuine land stewardship and corporate lip service to sustainable agriculture is one of the biggest challenges to transforming our respective food systems. The United States Department of Agriculture's definition of "sustainable agriculture" claims that it seeks to "increase profitable farm income, promote environmental stewardship, enhance quality of life for farm families and communities, and increase production for human food and fiber needs" (National Institute of Food and Agriculture 2025). The order of the four components in this definition is instructive—clearly, the government agency's focus is on profit. To be fair, if farms go out of business, farmers will not be able to grow food for human consumption, regardless of whether they are growing it sustainably. In the analysis that follows, I suggest ways to integrate western concepts of sustainable agriculture with Indigenous agricultural practices through holistic practices that value the ways in which agriculture can nourish both people and the Earth.

There are clear linkages between the concept of mālama ʻāina in Hawaiʻi and land stewardship in Aotearoa New Zealand. *Kaitiakitanga whenua* (protecting and nurturing the land) has the same basis in Māori genealogy as it does in Native Hawaiian creation stories. This guardianship of the land is inherent in Māori culture, and both Māori and Pākehā farmers and the food system advocates I interviewed rely on it. Some of their practices are based on a combination of western scientific agricultural knowledge infused with a Māori worldview, resulting in sustainable regenerative agricultural practices. For example, the PermaDynamics mother–daughter team of Frieda Lotz-Keegan and Ness Keegan "increased productivity by creating quite a complex yet complementary system of different elements through permaculture" (Lotz-Keegan 2020). Lotz-Keegan went on to provide an overview of the reasoning behind the PermaDynamics agricultural systems: "my heart's in regenerative agriculture and how I use syntropic food for our systems to really fast track succession and regenerate the land back into abundance and productivity. So that's kind of where my passion is" (2020). Although this would seem to be focused on productivity and, therefore, perhaps the economic value of certain crops, the larger narrative describes the ecosystem services provided by different plants and animals, and their impacts on waterway cleanliness and water retention in the soil to reduce water consumption. Similarly, Jessica Barnes's community market garden in urban Wellington uses organic and regenerative practices to ensure future success in food production for the surrounding urban community. The point is to bring in as few external inputs as possible and create a self-sustaining system.

These ideas are not new. They are based in Indigenous land management practices and have a history of success dating back millennia. Kate Cherrington explains that the genealogy of special Native plants relates back to being a guardian of the planet and "acknowledges multiple ways of being, knowing, and doing which puts it into a spiritual realm" (Cherrington 2020). She also articulates the story by way of using *whakapapa* (genealogy) as a verb, saying that we should "whakapapa the land back to the people, and if they can do that in a way that is caring and kind, that makes for a particular connection" (Cherrington 2020). Cathy Tait-Jameson, the owner of BioFarm, an organic dairy farm in Palmerston North that makes some of the best yogurt in Aotearoa New Zealand from happy pasture-raised and fed cows I was lucky enough to meet, also links her Māori heritage to ancestral ways of farming and thinking through biodynamic farming.

> I sort of discovered my Māori heritage a few years after we bought the farm from my husband's family. Looking at mythology and ancestral ways of farming and navigating and thinking, oh my goodness, this is also the biodynamic way. So really it just made us realize that it is just the natural way. So, this is how we farm, the way farming has been for most since the beginning. Whereas knowledge comes from here [pointing to her head and then heart], just taking everything that comes into your farm and into your head and applying it to your own ecosystem. (Tait-Jameson 2020)

Applying Rudolph Steiner's (1993) biodynamic principles of holistic ecological and ethical approaches to farming, gardening, nutrition, and food (Biodynamic Association 2024) was an easy extension of Tait-Jameson's understanding of her Māori ancestral farming practices.

Kate Walmsley's focus on composting is a part of this larger conversation as well. As the director of the composting arm of Kaicycle, an urban farm and community compost organization in the heart of Wellington, Aotearoa New Zealand, she says that we should be "framing composting as equally important. You cannot grow food regeneratively if we're not turning our urban waste streams into high quality compost" (Walmsley 2020). These practices are applicable in both rural and urban areas, at different scales of course, but just because they are occurring in an urban area like Wellington does not make them any less linked to Māori agricultural practices.

Finally, Angela Clifford further reinforced this point when talking about diversity—of crops and of perspectives. She told me that:

> An acceptance of diversity is super important. A diversity of perspectives, a diversity of voices. It's a reflection of the natural systems that we value. We're permaculturalists. The most successful natural systems are diverse. Permaculturalists are the systems-thinkers, so that's really important to me, is that there are people who

don't think like I do that you continue to bring into the conversation. And people
that challenge all of our thinking, that's super important as well. (Clifford 2020)

This view is precisely what traditional ecological knowledge is based on.
Whether one wants to assign the label of permaculture, regenerative agriculture,
or Indigenous agriculture, the result is the same. A focus on diversity of crops,
of ideas, and of systems is key to successful and sustainable agriculture that will
feed communities and regenerate the soil at the same time so that the ʻāina and
whenua can *keep* feeding people for future generations to come.

Feminist Political Ecology as Food System Praxis

Environmental activism through material practices is shaped by the situated knowledges and everyday experiences of the food system change agents interviewed in
this book. As Juanita Sundberg explains in her Feminist Political Ecology entry
for *The International Encyclopedia of Geography* (2017), FPE "demonstrates
how social identities are constituted in and through relations with nature and
every day material practices…connecting theory with praxis" (2). For example,
Claire Sullivan, currently the chief executive officer at Farm Link Hawaiʻi (by
way of leadership positions at MAʻO Farms, Whole Foods, and Maui Land and
Pineapple), explains that in her family, food was a way to enact values in the
world while understanding the social and environmental conditions of production. She recognizes her positionality as a woman from a family with the means
to make the kinds of food choices that supported their values and sees that this
privilege reproduces the problematic choice within a neoliberal capitalist system
that encourages us to "vote with our forks." In exploring the limits to her agency,
Sullivan saw that she could make a difference beyond her role as a consumer. Her
perspective of agriculture is that it shapes intersectionality as a practice, rather
than an identity category—from an even wider angle than we may be accustomed
to viewing it. She clarifies her perspective by sharing her work experiences at
both Maui Land and Pineapple and subsequently at Whole Foods:

> Increasingly, it became clear that agriculture was interesting because it was
> more of a space of intersection. Ecosystem health intersecting with individual
> human health alongside cultural well-being and economic vitality. There are all
> of the pieces for an incredibly fruitful space. There is a relevance in all of those
> spheres simultaneously and it became abundantly clear to me that agriculture is

really where it's at. You're thinking about a nexus between the human and natural world and [it] includes all these aspects within the human world. (Sullivan 2019)

Sullivan understands the natural world of ecosystem services and sustainable agriculture—that is, efforts to grow local food by local people and for local people on a relatable scale. Her view of intersectionality includes the positionality of the natural world in its meaning and resonates with Farhana Sultana and Andrea Nightingale's conceptualization of intersectionality, which considers how subject identity is constituted in and through material ecological relations (cited in Sundberg 2017) as well as looking toward how we can foster this kind of intersectional analysis when making decisions at both the individual and systemic levels.

None of this work is easy, nor is it simple. These stories demonstrate that much of the work is done out of passion for good, clean, and fair food with access for all. Nanette Geller's work running the electronic benefits transfer (EBT) program at several Hawaiʻi Farm Bureau farmers' markets exemplifies these important efforts to avoid the potential elitism of access to fresh whole foods. She explains that:

Social justice comes together with my lifelong passion for believing that everybody should be able to do well. Everyone should eat good food and good food means it has to be delicious and it has to be healthy, and it has to be environmentally safe. All of that has to come together. [I focus on] projects that will bring together this concept of really good, fresh local foods, not just produce but other local foods as well with people who might not have access, whether for financial reasons or for physical constraints. I want to know the quality and the freshness, but also the environmental and labor impacts. (Geller 2019)

Geller claims that her perspective on gender in the food system is influenced by her age, but she was, and continues to be, clearly ahead of her time. She grew up in the 1950s and 1960s, and

in those days, being defined as a woman meant you're going to get married and have children and be a homemaker and that was never going to be me. I was aware that this is the definition other people wanted from me, but I was not going to accept that definition. I learned to stand up for who I am because I don't let other people define me. (Geller 2019)

Defying expectations, she became a computer programmer and worked in New York and Japan. Her experiences as the only woman in the room paved the way for her willingness to think outside the box to bring EBT terminals to farmers' markets on Oʻahu so that people with Supplemental Nutrition Assistance Program (SNAP) benefits could buy fresh produce and other locally produced goods. This had already been done on the continent, but Hawaiʻi was lagging behind. Her programming skills led to a problem-solving mindset that enabled her to find ways to incorporate EBT terminals at the farmers' markets by having customers swipe their EBT cards at a centralized wireless terminal located at the market's information booth. Customers received farmers' market tokens in exchange for a portion of their SNAP benefit balance and could spend them on eligible foods at participating vendors.

Being self-sustaining, whether for a business or a nonprofit organization, is a central concern no matter its structure. For example, Jessica Barnes, the community garden manager of For The Better Good in Wellington explains that different structures work for different communities. Community gardens are typically places where people come to work on their own plots of land on publicly owned property. However, For The Better Good is

> not a community garden in the sense that community members have plots. It's a community garden in the sense that anyone is welcome into the space and can contribute. The food goes back into the Well-Fed kitchen, but it's also meant to be self-sustaining. Hospitality Wellington is buying our greens and veggies. The idea is to make it as self-sustaining as possible and also show it as a model that can be done, have it work, and be replicable. (Barnes 2020)

At another urban farm in Wellington, Kaicycle's vision is to have compost hubs around the city to collect food waste from residents, and turn it into compost.

> In the future, once we have more of these kind of compost hubs around the city, [we want to] focus on hubs to collect from the residents around it. It has to be a small area. You walk your food waste over weekly, and you come home with a free veggie box. And we'll explore how that model might look in the future. But accessibility always has to be a priority. So, with this collective, the idea is to have a central commons to share and build that knowledge base and invite people into the space to benefit from it. That's what we're doing for New Zealand. (Walmsley 2020)

The idea, in both instances, is to have a replicable model that can be used elsewhere while being self-sustaining for the individual organizations—economically, socially, and environmentally. Moreover, it is important for each model to be decentralized, so that it remains accessible to different communities and modifiable for their own needs and benefits. This is especially relevant for small-scale organizations working in urban food systems. As Walmsley describes, "really purposeful urban agriculture moves us toward a circular economy within food systems" (2020). This statement is exactly the kind of solutions-based perspective needed to disrupt the current food system and move it toward sustainability.

Some interviewees mentioned practical solutions based on incremental alterations that have broad implications for larger food system changes. For example, Barnes (2020) explained how current metrics are problematic in terms of measuring ecosystem health. The data collected tends to be in pounds of food, but she wondered what kind of other metrics might be more appropriate.

> I think the standard right now is "how many pounds of food are you producing?" Whereas there are other sorts of ecosystem services metrics that regenerative agriculture produces that are not measured in pounds of food. This is especially relevant in New Zealand with our waterways. That's a huge, huge issue that we're having here. There's no life left in the waterways just because of the livestock [and runoff] going into the waterways. (Barnes 2020)

Regenerative agriculture is key to improving ecosystem and, by extension, human health, but current data-collection practices privilege conventional agriculture, and are once again focused on short-term gains. There are different solutions to these challenges, whether they are related to policy, assessment, specific agricultural practices, or environmental sustainability, but they all focus on long-term food system change.

A food system transformation cannot occur without revising existing land management practices. The long plantation agriculture history of Hawaiʻi, which dates from the early part of the nineteenth century all the way to the very end of the twentieth century, means that almost two hundred years of extractive agriculture have decimated soil health and environmental quality. Part of the equation relates to a long-standing land-use policy that privileges large tracts of land concentrated into few owners. Indeed, as Claire Sullivan notes,

> In some ways, we're perpetuating the plantation model where we have this really steep hierarchy with very few well-paid individuals at the top with a sophisticated skill set but with laborers who are not invested in terms of their

skill set development and who are frankly exploited for a physical contribution. And when we talk about our post-plantation future, we get really caught up in a war. How are we going to deal with the land? The land is still all land banked and we have too many big landholders or what are we gonna do about the water cisterns? You know, it used to be the plantations that facilitated the upkeep of irrigation systems. Those are all really important questions. But we aren't having that conversation about people's role. (Sullivan 2019)

Although land tenure and ownership structures are slowing changing in Hawai'i, system-level changes must occur prior to any real food system overhauls. The impetus behind some of these changes are rooted both in Indigenous scientific information and the discussion around regenerative agriculture, an approach to land management that encompasses all aspects of agriculture through a network of "entities who grow, enhance, distribute, and consume goods and services-instead of a linear supply chain…to restore soil and ecosystem health, address inequity, and leave our land, waters, and climate in better shape for future generations" (Natural Resources Defense Council 2021). The focus on future generations is taken directly from traditional ecological knowledge; to the Natural Resources Defense Council's credit, they acknowledge that these are not new ideas and have been part of Indigenous agricultural systems for millennia. A holistic understanding of agriculture includes human relationships with ecosystems as well as with each other, echoing the intersectional FPE approach discussed earlier. It re-regionalizes food systems to bring them back from large-scale, industrialized systems designed for economies of scale, but not for soil and human health and well-being. Smaller-scale agriculture fosters community-building. As Sullivan shared:

The most gratifying part of my [Whole Foods] experience was hearing from producers that Whole Foods had a catalytic role for the system. My hope was that Whole Foods with its, at that point, one store and then two and then three, was going to change the system, but that it could be catalytic for how others would participate in the system. Producers told me that the kinds of conversations they were having with other retailers and grocery buyers were transformed from one year to the next. And we talked about local food systems and generating community-based food systems. And it was at least catalytic, it was important. But it's very critical now that the torch be passed to others who are willing to be the leaders in that space who don't have the same set of constraints. (Sullivan 2019)

Sullivan's work shows that working within the capitalist system to foster change has both potential and serious limitations. She understands the role of humans within the ecosystem and sustainable agriculture, and how that expands the scope of intersectional praxis. However, the fact that at both Maui Land and Pineapple and Whole Foods, the leadership was beholden to board members as well as shareholders looking to increase their profits meant that Sullivan was limited by the constraints of the corporate capitalist system. Sullivan tried to prevent her work from being co-opted but realized that the systemic forces at play could not sustain her goals. In Hawaiʻi, she was one of the only interviewees to attempt to effect change by working through a for-profit business; most of the others worked either through legislative means or with nonprofit organizations to support AFNs. In Aotearoa New Zealand, three women I interviewed on the North Island— Jenny Lux, owner of Lux Organics, a five-acre organic farm in Rotorua; Cathy Tait-Jameson, owner of BioFarm (one of the earliest organic dairies there); and Kay Baxter, the doyenne of seed saving—were all attempting to use a sustain-ability-based business model to thrive within the existing capitalist framework.

Working within the capitalist system to foster change is one way to go about addressing problems within the food system, but the neoliberal capitalist system inherently privileges industrialized foods. If we consider the colonial histories of Hawaiʻi and Aotearoa New Zealand discussed in Chapter 1, then the systemic complications within the food system become incredibly difficult to overcome. Some of the respondents argued that bypassing the for-profit model altogether by working through cooperative systems was more likely to result in lasting change. Laurie Carlson, one of the founders of Kokua Food Market, the longest running food cooperative on the island of Oʻahu, claims that the current structural problems with the food system are in fact supported by government:

> Corporations are making all kinds of messes and the governments are really supporting their model. Underlying all of these challenges is a food system that subsidizes the wrong things. Why don't we have subsidies on organic produce, which is reducing carbon, instead of opting for industrial corn? The underlying structure is so wrong. It's just so wrong. (Carlson 2019)

Understanding and problematizing food security's western focus on capitalist free-market solutions is central to Indigenous and gendered food sovereignty discourse. In fact, even though it includes state action, which can have its own attendant problems and has done violence to Indigenous and marginalized groups in the past, food system transformation cannot be accomplished without policy and legislative processes. Reclaiming regional and sustainable food systems must be supported by government action and political will prior to the implementation of any free-market strategies, simply because it is unlikely that the market will move away from the focus on short-term profits without any incentives to do so. These could be based on low-interest agricultural loans or tax breaks for growing diversified crops using regenerative agricultural practices, for example.

> We have no leadership on a national level. We have a little bit on the international level, but not much on the local level. There was a new chapter in the Hawai'i Revised Statutes for the incorporation of consumer cooperatives. We did it by working with all these other cooperatives, housing, credit unions and reporting requirements. (Carlson 2019)

Carlson encountered challenges in setting up the structure for the cooperative model's success. Kokua Market ran into financial difficulties in 2018 when the remodeling of a high-rise in the area blocked access to its store, and it has struggled to regain its financial footing. Carlson was elected chairperson of the board to try to turn things around. The store operated on and off until 2024, when it closed for good. She views the lack of government support as a critical stumbling block for local food system sustainability.

Sustainable Agriculture

Sustainable agriculture is an integral part of a healthy community food system. Nowhere is this truer than in an archipelago, where a closed loop system thrived for hundreds of years prior to contact with European colonizers. The narratives in this project connect sustainable agriculture to education and acknowledge the importance of incorporating sustainable ecological principles into attitudes toward land and the environment. These perspectives are guided by a general understanding of abundance and growth through regenerative rather than extractive means. Some of the stories reflect an understanding of sustainable agriculture as it relates to state agriculture policies, and others share practical aspects of sustainable agriculture to ensure a wide dissemination of knowledge.

The women's stories consistently express the value of relationships and networks, both to the land and to the people. For example, Claire Sullivan credits her mother for instilling in her the value of sustainable agriculture as a "space that's generative of community well-being" (Sullivan 2019). Creating that space in community affords us the time to really listen and understand how weaving land and people together creates a larger narrative that exemplifies the importance of the work. Industrialized agriculture is one of the single leading causes of climate change, accounting for 10% of carbon emissions in the United States alone (Environmental Protection Agency 2022). This is not news to most of the respondents. Indeed, Meleana Judd's parents ran a solar energy company, so she already knew that "agriculture is just as much a contributor to climate change as energy…so I decided I had to be involved in agriculture" (Judd 2019). Due to her family's experience, as well as her mission to get involved with sustainable agriculture by starting a small community farm on the North Shore of Oʻahu, Judd also saw how important policy is to the success of small sustainable farm ventures. She knows how important strong relationships are to the surrounding community. To that end, Waihuena Farm has hosted permaculture courses, community yoga classes, art classes for children, free concerts, and once-a-month potlucks. However, Judd claims that the farm is still not economically sustainable to stand on its own. Part of the problem, she asserts, is that there is little to no support from the state for this kind of agriculture.

> It's just crazy when you look at the stuff, when our Department of Agriculture has what percent? Zero point one percent of the budget? I wonder, like, "hello, we all eat every day. We're in the middle of the Pacific. This is ridiculous." When I used to attend the soil water conservation district meetings, just for a while, I wanted to know: how does agriculture work here? I went to Farm Bureau meetings for a while too. And I just hit that model every time: very low wages and extremely large production. (Judd 2019)

That lack of support and political will leads to continued reliance on imported food, as does the Hawaiʻi Department of Agriculture's perpetuation of the large-scale, plantation model of agriculture as the only feasible way to farm for a profit. This buys into the neocolonial system, whereby many of the landowners are corporations with seats on the continent or even foreign countries. This is not the case for all large tracts of land, yet it is an important factor in the way agriculture is structured in Hawaiʻi. This model does not suggest any kind of relationship to the land or to the people working it, beyond exploitative labor for corporate profits. Judd herself explains that her relationship to agriculture started when she was a child—foraging for fruit in the neighborhood, for example, and the initial joy and inspiration of having access to the abundance from ʻāina. She understands her privilege, since she acknowledges that many of her friends did not have access to that abundance, but she also rejoices in the experience and the way it forged her life path toward appreciating the land's bounty.

The stories in this project innovatively reimagine what Daniela Spoto, the Director of Food Equity at the Hawaiʻi Appleseed Center for Law and Economic Justice, which works to change systems that perpetuate inequality through research and advocacy, calls the "production space," while honoring Indigenous ways of knowing and acknowledging and valuing the scientific basis of Native agricultural practices. This "best of both worlds" approach can be found through the narratives' consideration of agroecological principles as well as regenerative agriculture. These useful applications of land-use practices show the amount of care and respect the women have for what sustainable agriculture can bring to communities. For instance, Kuʻulei Samson, from Hoa ʻĀina O Mākaha on the Leeward Coast of Oʻahu, explains that we are all meant to be farmers because we need food to survive. Growing that food means understanding the cycles of life, ecosystem services, and the judicious use of compost—just as it did to Native planters—but it also means growing relationships by sharing food with our neighbors, families, and friends when we have too much. Alternatively, it means composting the extra produce so that it comes back as nutrients to give seeds their next lives (Samson 2020). She also shares that this cycle not only reflects regenerative ecological principles from both a western perspective and an Indigenous one, insofar as the former is informed by the latter, but also fosters community and love. She has seen the community members she works with growing food for their community:

> To find that love and feel that love and realize that that love came from them and they're just going right back in a cycle, it's hard to stop. It's kind of addicting. A lot of it is experiments and when they start to experiment on their own, they kind of find their little comfort zone (Samson 2020)

Similarly, Cole shares that her journey to this work started when the Kohala Center started to focus on energy independence and ecosystem health (Cole 2019) when no one was interested in changing the status quo except for a group of strong and committed women who could see that reliance on imported foods was an unsustainable model for feeding communities in Hawaiʻi. Through prior education in cultural anthropology and archeology, she and others like Lehn Huff on Maui focused on the relationships between land and people in an island environment, especially as it affects Indigenous populations. The land became alive for them (Huff 2019) both as a source of food and as a source of stories and abundance within Kanaka Maoli genealogies. Correspondingly, in developing countries, women do the bulk of the labor in agricultural production and trade, and as Pimbert (2009) explains, they are mostly responsible for feeding their families whereas their husbands tend to be concerned with cash or export crops. This means that "women have specific, but unrecognized, traditional knowledge of seeds, harvesting and storage techniques and traditional products" (8). This "women's knowledge" resonates with Indigenous agricultural and ecological knowledge, and often, the two are one and the same. These traditions and practices tend to be passed down orally through the generations, and although they are generally ignored and undervalued by modern agricultural practices, they seem to be making some inroads as tools in the fight against climate change through sustainable agriculture.

Ensuring that the relationship between land and environment can foster a healthy food system is the primary concern. Huambachano (2019) shows that the Food and Agriculture Organization aims to foster economic viability, provide benefits for all members of society, and improve ecosystems in its definition of sustainable food systems. Sarah Smuts-Kennedy is an artist and biodynamic gardener based an hour north of Auckland. She founded an organization called For the Love of Bees to promote safe spaces for pollinators, people, and the planet. Her work is wide ranging in terms of its vision(s), but her focus on combining art and bees within urban areas is another way to measure the connection between land and environmental conditions. She asserts that bees are an indicator of ecosystem health:

> It's not about bees so much as it is about the environment. Bees are like the canary in the coal mine. They are an indicator of ecosystem well-being. When they are flying three kilometers, that's a three-kilometer radius project. So if we have bees, we want to be making sure the three-kilometer radius around those bees are safe for bees. What is safe for bees? For example, things that aren't safe for bees are lack of foraging habitat, pesticides, insecticides, herbicides, and fungicides. It is a fantastic way to start talking about regenerative agriculture. In essence, transformation occurs by making things visible. (Smuts-Kennedy 2020)

Her art installations, beehives, and garden boxes in urban settings have inspired both acclamation and ire. Some Māori community members told her, rightly, that her work was contributing to gentrification of certain urban areas because it replicates similar projects in upscale neighborhoods. She told me that she was working on understanding her privilege in this space. She explained that "we built [the Māori designed] art creation and we looked at what land loss meant to urban Māori. We used the site as a space to talk about land loss and what that means in regard to being able to look after oneself" (Smuts-Kennedy 2020). This work to understand privilege extends to the larger For the Love of Bees organization and remains an important guiding principle in the work they do by uplifting others, and amplifying the art and work of marginalized communities, especially in urban Auckland. Indeed, they use their platform to call policymakers' attention to this work by placing the art installations and gardens quite literally at the bottom of city and state government buildings.

Cathy Tait-Jameson's work in the organic dairy industry with BioFarm (their yogurt is incredible) is a testament to the work of lifting up land ethic practices, in this case from her Māori ancestors. She views it as an opportunity to give back to her community and her heritage at the same time.

> And for me, it was to give an opportunity for Māori growers to validate what they're doing. It was not about ticking the boxes and adhering to rules. It was about the story of the food and the provenance of it and why it was grown by the people. Which to me is far more relevant when you are actually working the land. You want to be able to tell your story. You don't want to just tick the box. More and more the auditors come. They flap up their laptops and they talk the whole time. They don't even make eye contact. And it takes away from the importance of what you're doing. You know, you want some relief to be able to share with someone who's really interested in why you do this every day. (Tait-Jameson 2020)

How do we combat these disconnected attitudes between what is valued by policymakers and bureaucrats, and pivot toward a more holistic view of agriculture? Once again, turning to Indigenous values is instructive. Kay Baxter shares the following:

> There is a critical importance of reconnection to our food, to land, and the place where we live. We've got to create a new culture because our ancestors were totally connected to the places they lived and grew food. Now, we've got different land, different places, and different foods. We kind of have to recreate the food that grows where we live. We have to regenerate ecological health. Water. Health. Food. Human health. Everything has to be regenerated. The only way to do that is by reconnecting everything up again because it's all been disconnected. (Baxter 2020)

This turn toward reconnection has deep roots in many Indigenous communities, but also in immigrant and marginalized communities. Angela Clifford of Eat New Zealand says that "we recognized really early on that wines have the sense of terroir or the Māori word is *tūrangawaewae*—this idea of a place to be from and its connection to the Earth and its environment. So, of course, that makes sense from a food perspective as well" (Clifford 2020). This pivot toward a more connected food system is precisely what Rangimārie Mules called for when she said that we need to get back to our roots and become the masters of our own local contexts and environments to become key players in our own systems at home (Mules 2020). Decentralizing production, distribution, and consumption of food is key to fostering food system health and sustainability in the long-term.

Land Stewardship–Hawaiʻi's Mālama ʻĀina

To decentralize our food system, we must re-regionalize it. This will enable us to regain a connection with the surrounding land. Clearly, colonialism has had the most drastic impact on Native peoples, separating them from their ancestral lands and connections to ancestral knowledges and foodways. However, reconnecting with the land has a potentially beneficial impact on just about everyone. If we are going to take the threats of climate change seriously (which we should have already been doing for the last three decades), it behooves us to understand how land and people can interact sustainably to feed ourselves and reduce carbon emissions at the same time. Once again, valuing Indigenous knowledge regarding land stewardship is an ideal place to start. The most effective way to move toward climate resilience and sustainable food access for everyone would be to listen to *kūpuna* (elders) and community members who know and understand microclimates, and who respect agroecological principles rooted in spiritual practices that value different aspects of ecosystems. Dr. Summer Maunakea, a professor of Education at the University of Hawaiʻi at Mānoa (UH Mānoa), calls this a "genealogy of knowledge about growing that comes from kūpuna all over" (Maunakea 2019).

Nancy Redfeather, an expert seed saver and the former Kū ʻĀina Pā Education program director at the Kohala Center on Hawaiʻi Island, explains that these goals are not without their challenges:

> You've got family members or people who lost their connection completely
> to the land. And so, it's up to us and the future generations to bring it back, to

make that connection more evident. Here in Hawaiʻi, we really have the perfect environment and the perfect kind of isolated situation to fight for that to happen, but it's been difficult mainly because of the land situation. We have never been able to break up these large land trusts that we have everywhere. And there was a really good attempt at that in the 1990s. There was a year-long meeting in Honolulu with all of those landowners, to see if the state could come up with some kind of plan to move on that just because they were trying to fulfill the 1978 constitutional amendment, Article 13, which states that you should protect and preserve agricultural land. (Redfeather 2019)

The Hawaiʻi state 1978 Constitutional Convention's Article 13 preserves land for agricultural use in perpetuity. This was definitely a step in the right direction and has been effective in preventing development on prime agricultural land—for the most part. Yet developers are a canny bunch and are willing to wait out land-use zoning changes to build homes on formerly productive agricultural parcels. As with most desirable places to live on the continent, a serious housing crisis afflicts Hawaiʻi and there is political will to build more single-family homes in order to prevent a brain drain—whereby the adult children of Hawaiʻi residents are forced to move to places with a cheaper cost of living on the continent, perhaps after attending college there, due to the lack of on-island housing and employment opportunities beyond tourism. For example, the Koa Ridge development on Oʻahu took more than fifteen years to receive its final zoning change, enduring long and costly litigation (Leone 2006; Shapiro 2013), and infrastructure such as roads, sewers, plumbing, and of course homes, are being built as of this writing. Oʻahu is in a particularly difficult position due to its dense population of around a million people, according to the 2020 Census, limited availability of land on an island, and the influx of anywhere between just over 6 million visitors in pre-pandemic 2019 to just under 6 million visitors by the end of 2024 on Oʻahu alone (Hawaiʻi Tourism Authority 2025).

On Hawaiʻi Island, the local food scene is much more developed. When asked how Hawaiʻi Island was so much further along than the other islands, Kristin Albrecht, the executive director of The Food Basket, the Hawaiʻi Island food bank, joked:

everybody always says that. But I think it's simply that we have a lot of land and a lot of disasters that throw us together really closely and also really keep that urgency at the top of our radar. There's nothing like death from a chronic disease that's totally avoidable through nutrition to sort of wake one up, you know? (Albrecht 2019)

While Albrecht was clearly being facetious, she does signal that with every challenge, there is an opportunity. Indeed, Kuʻulei Samson sees the relationship with the land differently, yet with a similar goal. She told me that the land doesn't discriminate. No matter our "shape, size or color, anyone can grow food because it's about healing ourselves" (Samson 2020). Samson's narrative about healing can be interpreted in two ways: first, we can heal our bodies with healthy food, and second, we can heal our spirits through a connection with the land. Her background as a Hawaiian Studies major, her long-time work at MAʻO Farms, and subsequently at Hoʻa ʻĀina O Mākaha indicates that the second part is just as important as the first part—they cannot be separated, and the latter contributes significantly to the former.

Gardening, perhaps with their own relatives, is one of the ways several of the women interviewed for this book, have come to value their connections with the land, as well as growing, cooking, and eating good food. Numerous participants identified gardening with their mothers as a definitive moment in their lives. Rachel Ladrig, formerly at Kahumana Organic Farm and Food Hub and now a farm coach on the Windward side of Oʻahu for GoFarm Hawaiʻi, did not grow up around farming, but her mom had a garden, and it was one of the only ways that they connected. Some of her fondest memories were in the garden at her neighbor's house and at her grandma's (Ladrig 2019). Similarly, Meleana Judd had a mother who gardened and fostered her initial connection with land. Summer Maunakea fought against bureaucratic obstacles at the university to grow a garden to teach her pre-service teachers how to incorporate gardening into their curriculum. However, she came to it the same way as the others, starting what she called a "trial and error" garden with her parents at the family's home in Waipahu to improve their nutrition and health outcomes, and to learn how to grow food so that she could turn around and teach her students effectively. The ability to grow something from seed, care for it, see it grow, take it out of the ground, and eat it is a priceless journey, and it's one of the biggest draws for many of the participants who either garden themselves or teach others (adults or children) how to garden. Facilitating that process is gratifying in and of itself, but the fact that the positive outcomes extend to families and communities is an added bonus. Kukui Maunakea-Forth, a founding member of the Waiʻanae Re-development Corporation and executive director of MAʻO Farms, explains that their interns are allowed and indeed encouraged to take home any leftover produce after working at the farm and/or the farmers' markets. The farm is currently hosting a large-scale study through the John A. Burns School of Medicine at UH Mānoa to determine whether this dissemination of fresh, and in MAʻO's case, organic produce has beneficial nutritional and health outcomes for the interns' families. Maunakea-Forth's nephew, Dr. Alika Maunakea, is leading the study, "Socioecological Determinants of Immunoepigenetic Signatures of Diabetes Risk in Indigenous Communities," which was awarded a National Institutes of Health (NIH) five-year grant of US$3.3 million[2] (Hawai'i Social Epigenomics Early Diabetes Cohort 2021). Understanding social factors that influence health outcomes is key to this project. Kaui Sana, the farm manager at MA'O Farms, sees the impacts firsthand. She asks herself:

> How can we create those experiences for everybody when we're sharing space here? When they present in school and they get help from one of us, it's the whole systems-thinking and change in how to heal and strengthen community. And I'm really happy that food is a big part of that, because for a lot of families, we've lost our connection to food. Knowing what we put in our mouth and into our family's mouth is probably one of most powerful things we can do in in changing systems and changing choices that we can make. Planting food, some people might not take it as deep as others, but some people will get the deeper meaning. There is a fair amount of families here on welfare. For them to have that kind of access to that kind of food is definitely one of our missions to really try and push all of our food out. Any extra veggies here, the students take home. We don't charge them. We want them to give it to their families and to their aunties, uncles, or grandmas. (Sana 2019)

This circular system of giving food to their interns' families is now part of the medical school study, but it has been a long-standing practice at MA'O Farms. When their production capacity was relatively low, the farm was criticized for selling to high-end restaurants in Honolulu instead of ensuring that the food they grew stayed in their surrounding community on the Leeward Coast. Now that their land base has expanded dramatically (from the originally leased 5 acres to a total of 237 acres now in production), they are able to distribute food more equitably and reach their community through increased farmers' market venues, because there are now two consistent farmers' markets on the Leeward Coast.

In Hawai'i, local food production has ebbed and flowed in terms of both capacity and demand for the past several decades. The COVID-19 pandemic certainly increased demand and interest in climate-change resilience and related

---

[2.] Continued funding is uncertain due to federal funding cuts implemented in 2025.

disaster preparedness. After the plantation era, the Hawai'i Regional Cuisine (HRC) movement fostered awareness of how to champion local production, but as Claire Sullivan says, it was

> super rarefied, enduringly very elite, very low volume, high value. It then shifted in the early 2000s to farmers' markets, so there started to be a slight democratization of access and telling of stories with all the tourists. But there was this moment right away, around 2004 to 2010, that was our heyday for farmers' markets. There was this widening of market access for farms, and they were feeling like they could grow more things and could grow more volume. They didn't have to have a relationship with Alan Wong or Roy [Yamaguchi—two famous HRC chefs]. Maybe they could go beyond that. I gave presentations at that point in time, and it was like "OK, the next step is groceries. This is where we go now." This is really exciting because most people shop at the grocery store. They don't shop at the farmer's market. If we want to genuinely link up local production and local consumption, the grocery store is the natural place to do it. And I would get all excited about that and talk about how that was the next step in the evolution. The grocery store space was unfolding, but the next step that I would get really keen to explore was institutional purchasing, like schools and hospitals. (Sullivan 2019)

The relationship between increased local food production and public and environmental health is key here. Daniela Spoto, from the Hawai'i Appleseed Center for Law and Economic Justice, mentions the available evidence of that connection and adds the additional layer of economic development as well. She explains that this is the triple bottom line that links public health, environmental sustainability, and economic development in the following way:

> The way that we marketed the Double [Up Food] Bux program was as a triple bottom line. We called it a triple win for families, farmers, and the economy. For the families, it's really the health argument and how this is going to make our communities healthy. That includes families and residents. It's gonna be better for local farmers who are going to grow local food production, to make an impact based on the environmental argument. And then for the economy, keeping capital circulating in the local community is important. If you're a farmer, you're not necessarily going to say that "my goal is to make my community healthier." You can see that because it's important, but you might be more interested in your bottom line. So that one goal, I think, is actually a triple goal. We all need to

make sure that any solution we find addresses all of those things in order to get
everybody on board. (Spoto 2019)

Identifying these three separate goals while showing their interdependence is a
critical part of Spoto's role in supporting food system change. Her work and that
of the other women in the project bridge a variety of ideas. For example, Rachel
Ladrig expresses it as her way of being of service, to genuinely build relationships and being the connecting fabric that weaves people, projects, and ideas
together. Sana views her work as part of community healing, and Samson sees it
as fostering human well-being through working with the land. Geller worked to
provide practical changes to serve SNAP recipients at farmers' markets. Maunakea
teaches pre-service teachers how to include ʻāina in their lesson plans. Shapiro
created a cooperative of ʻulu growers to bring awareness and attention back to
an almost forgotten staple crop. Albrecht makes sure underserved people have
access to fresh local foods. Tait-Jameson and Lux run successful and sustainable
organic farms. These are just a few of the women encountered in this chapter
who are working to change the food system, whether incrementally in their own
regions, or on a larger scale, throughout an entire state. Seen through the lens
of Spoto's three goals, they all demonstrate a powerful purpose in addressing
food system change.

The relationship between food and family cannot be separated from love of the
land or from the violence done to Kanaka Maoli and Māori through colonialism
that underlies many of the narratives. Nurturing and loving through sharing
food cannot be accomplished if there is no land upon which to grow food in the
first place. The non-Indigenous women in this study understand their respective
roles in settler colonial society, as do I. For example, Lehn Huff studied anthropology and archeology, where she discovered that learning about the land
brought it alive for her and that all of the issues in an island environment affect
Indigenous peoples due to colonization (Huff 2019). She attained this knowledge
through formal education, as did Frankie Koethe. However, Koethe learned that
community groups were an invaluable source of knowledge, not only about
agriculture and issues surrounding land stewardship, but more specifically in
revealing how women interacted within the settler colonial space in trying to
make a living and feed their respective communities at the same time. In both
instances, they understood colonial oppressions and do important allyship work
to uplift and amplify the voices of food system actors, whether they are people
of color, Indigenous people, or immigrant farmers. Understanding this history
is critical to achieving what Daniela Spoto identifies as key: "we want to find

solutions that are going to completely disrupt the status quo and create equality and ensure community resilience. Island mentality is key here" (Spoto 2019). This takes us back to Hauʻofa's vision of a "sea of islands," because that idea necessitates stewardship and sustainability to foster resilience.

Conclusion

Nourishing soil leads to growing nutritious food to foster healthy communities. Connecting land stewardship based on traditional ecological knowledge and agroecological practices for sustainable agricultural production is key to fostering a regional food system that values AFNs. Instead of calling them "alternative" food networks, the goal is for that alterity to become the norm. The industrial agro-food system is not easily going to let go of its grasp of corporate profits, but women in this study are making inroads to reshape food systems in Hawaiʻi and Aotearoa New Zealand.

The practical solutions described in this chapter are among a few that address very specific problems, and while they are focused on a particular decolonized land ethic of stewardship, guardianship, and conservation, that emphasis extends to the food justice aspect of getting healthy food access to everyone. Stewardship is not only premised on a relationship between land and humans, but among humans caring for each other and invoking connections that will enable good, clean, and fair food to end up on people's plates everywhere.

CHAPTER 3

Education and Social Justice–Generational Food System Transformation

"'A 'ohe pau ka 'ike ka hālau ho 'okahi." / All knowledge is not taught in the same school—one can learn from many sources.
—Mary Kawena Pukui (1983)

Hands Turned to the Soil: Learning by Doing

Growing food and healthy communities at the same time is a lofty goal that starts with education. Through programs like those found under the auspices of the Hawai'i Farm-to-School and School Garden Hui, Lydi Morgan-Bernal gets kids outside and connected with nature and teaches them how to grow and eat the products of their labor. She explains that one of the Hawai'i Department of Education's "Five Promises" is equity. School gardens help students who might learn differently to thrive.

> If you want real equity, then you have to accommodate the fact that everyone learns differently and the kids that just don't do well in class are typically the stars of the garden because they're the most engaged. I even think things like homelessness and other social issues come from people not having a chance to get connected with something they care about at a young age and just giving up or checking out. Gardening and 'āina-based education are so foundational. It's about connecting kids to what matters so that they know what's most important. (Morgan-Bernal 2020)

Morgan-Bernal spent the formative years of her career as a garden educator herself. She has seen firsthand how turning children's hands to the 'āina and the soil impacts their attitudes toward learning and understanding of environmental issues.

I even see the progress we've made in the last 10 plus years. It seems that we're starting to put the pieces together for the food system. Things have been in disrepair, that was my impression in terms of how hard it is just to get local food into the schools. But what I like about farm-to-school is that it's not just getting the food onto the plate by involving the kids and all the amazing education that goes with that, but it's also getting them to grow it, so they understand that aspect of it, which inspires them to eat it. They eat whatever they grow. It is also about getting them out to farms, like farm field trips. It's doing chef demonstrations, looking at waste reduction through composting. What I love about this program is using gardens as outdoor classrooms. It's so much bigger than just the food that we eat and learning about our food systems. (Morgan-Bernal 2020)

Morgan-Bernal makes the connection between children growing fresh healthy food on school campuses and being willing to eat the products of their labor. Picky eaters are abundant in K–6 settings, where most of the Hawai'i farm-to-school education occurs, and enabling children to discover foods they might have otherwise refused is a feat.

The DOE identified two different communities to pilot this in and they were able to dedicate funding for two Farm-to-School coordinators. They are junior extension agents for the community in Wai'anae and Moloka'i and then Department of Health SNAP-ed program sent funds to match the funding so that the positions can be full time with some operating funds which is intriguing because this means it is fully state funded, and it's doing the work that we know needs to happen, which is someone to network school and community resources. You know, all the pieces that make up the community and support the three elements of the school which are school gardening, education, and food improvement. (Morgan-Bernal 2020)

The policy and lobbying aspects of the Farm-to-School and School Garden Hui's work is invaluable. Their insistence on asking the legislature to find funding for agricultural extension agents within the Hawai'i Department of Education is a testament to their tenacity and creativity. Normally, extension agents are funded through a combination of university and US Department of Agriculture (USDA) money, but neither of these entities were fully forthcoming with funding, so the Farm-to-School and School Garden Hui found another way to apportion the funding to deliver these two key positions to support healthy school food and garden education throughout the state.

We got the green light from the Department of Ed and Food Services to make a garden cafeteria program. So we're learning about what it takes to successfully communicate between the garden program and the cafeteria and to talk about "what do you want? How much of it? When do you need it?" But we actually worked out with school food that the garden programs will get paid for their produce. (Morgan-Bernal 2020)

It has taken more than a decade to institute these programs within the DOE and to ensure regular communication and networking among school garden educators. Nancy Redfeather's work through the Kohala Center, Lehn Huff's work on Maui, and Kōkua Hawai'i Foundation's entire mission (also a nonprofit run entirely by women), which reaches all of the islands, are precursors to this achievement. The fact that it has finally come to pass speaks to the determination of the women who made it happen. The state of Hawai'i has not been as responsive in introducing these changes to the school food system as other states on the continent. For instance, California has been a leader in sustainable school food programs, starting with the high-profile Edible Schoolyard, founded in 1995 by Chef Alice Waters in Berkeley, California. This movement was extended to a national level with Michelle Obama's "Let's Move" program, instituted in 2012. In Hawai'i, part of this unresponsiveness has to do with the unwieldy state bureaucracy; the Hawai'i state DOE is one entity that oversees 295 public and charter schools with over 168,000 children on seven islands (hawaiipublicschools.org 2022). This means there is one office for School Food Services for all the islands. At a school food policy meeting I attended in 2015 at the Hawai'i state capitol with a range of nonprofit executives, lawmakers, community organizers, and scholars submitting ideas about healthy school food, then-director Glenna Owens said that School Food Services' modus operandi was "what we do for one school, we have to do for all schools." There had not been an opportunity to pilot different school food projects until the most recent legislative win highlighted in Morgan-Bernal's narrative.

School gardens are not the only spaces where knowledge is shared among community. Before Nanette Geller's work to accept SNAP benefits at O'ahu farmers' markets, Alicia Higa had access to electricity and internet (the Wai'anae Coast Comprehensive Health Center [WCCHC] farmers' market was on the health center campus rather than a parking lot), so she was able to accept EBT cards to provide access to fresh, locally grown foods for low-income people in the area.

So last year we doubled over ninety thousand dollars of stock at our farmers' market on locally sourced items. This year, we're on target to do over one hundred

twenty-eight thousand dollars with the doubling [double SNAP bucks]. Our farmers'
markets are meant to be for food access, but also community gathering places to
get education, whether it's cultural education, sustainability education, or nutrition
education. We do large community events like our "Eat Local Challenge." It's
a month-long event that challenges our community to support local and really
make conscious decisions when they're doing their shopping and preparing their
menus. We do cooking demonstrations and sustainability activities. It's just a
month-long time with tons of education. (Higa 2019)

The markets at the WCCHC do more than just provide access to good food; they
provide education about healthy foods, seasonality of ingredients, culturally relevant foods, and Indigenous foodway traditions, and at the same time, they feed
dollars directly back into local farmers' pockets to encourage their sustainable
growing practices.

People are able to taste the food and then utilize their double [SNAP] bucks. We
have a price on it. It is really easy for people to make those decisions because
it wasn't costing them too much. If you're on a limited income and you have to
pay full price for things sometimes you don't want to choose something that's
new because if it gets wasted, that's resources wasted, right? So we have the "Eat
Local Challenge." We do a two-day event called Mauka to Makai that teaches our
community about where our water comes from, the traditional farming practices.
We also push food preparation, but we connect that on day one. We're up at
the farm teaching our community and we feed them almost 100 percent locally
sourced lunch from Wai'anae. It opens with traditional protocol between cultural
activities. All of it is focused around nutrition aspects, sustainability, culture. So
that theme is common throughout every single activity or workshop that we put
on. We also do monthly wellness workshops here at the health center that are
based on one of those three topics. (Higa 2019)

Throughout the farmers' market venue, educational stations and traditional
protocols explain how sustainable agriculture practices are tied to Indigenous
concepts like the Native Hawaiian ahupua'a land management system and the
importance of healthy watersheds to Indigenous farming practices. Additionally,
several of the respondents in Aotearoa New Zealand expressed their view that
community gardens, mostly run or maintained by women, are also spaces of
connection. Pounamu Skelton, an instructor in the Hua Parakore program in

Taranaki on the southwestern coast of the North Island, and Trish Allen, the founder of Rainbow Valley Farm in Matakana, both located in Aotearoa New Zealand, saw gardens as good places to grow relationships (2020). Allen started her community garden with a friend in 2012.

> I didn't really know if it would be a success. But it has been an enormous success. Everyone pitches in. It's all commonly owned. And we share the produce at the end of each session. Also, it's a little resource for the community. We've got a little stall and we've got a notice up there that if people want to harvest, that's okay. But please leave us something. Either some coins in the little box we've got, or some food scraps for our compost or some seaweed for our compost or whatever. You know, we're asking for a contribution. So it's not free and there's something expected in return. But it doesn't have to be money. (Allen 2020)

Allen's small community garden is a space to grow food, but also to make connections and to grow community based on sharing abundance, and not necessarily expecting monetary gain from it. Rather, she explains that "paying" with in-kind donations is totally acceptable and it bypasses the monetary economy altogether. She also acknowledges that sometimes people cannot afford to pay, and they take produce home regardless. She figures they need the food more than she does.

> It's women spearheading these garden and waste reduction efforts. The other thing is that waste is such a huge contributor to climate change so by wasting less and diverting waste, utilizing it, and reusing it, we're taking climate action. That's what the young people want. Climate action now. So by doing this work with waste, anybody can take climate action. Making that connection so people see it. I think it's really important. (Allen 2020)

Allen's view that the garden should be valued through contributions echoes several respondents who assigned worth to the work and products of community labor, using the community garden as an educational space, and even going beyond sharing skills and knowledge. They place their work within a larger context of waste reduction and climate action. Coming from yet another perspective on garden education, Skelton argued that not all knowledge is learned in a class-room. Experiential or hands-on learning means finding ways to learn how to be vulnerable with each other and support each other, by using the garden itself as a tool for change (Skelton 2020). Jessica Barnes explained a variety of uses for urban gardens, all for the community's benefit:

> There's all these parcels of urban places that are not serving their purpose any-more, but can be turned into something that is very abundant and fruitful and beneficial to the community. The next iteration of this garden is continuing to kind of finish up the garden because it's so new. We only really planted in October and continue to expand and then [we are] creating kind of child friendly spaces as well as wild spaces in terms of a lizard garden to support lizard populations here. We want to create a kind of safe space for the lizards to create habitat and then in turn, they'll eat our slugs that love our mulch. We're trying to support as much as we can the native wildlife that's around here. (Barnes 2020)

Barnes's urban community garden is a former bowling green in the heart of Wellington, Aotearoa New Zealand. It had been unused for some time and suffered from com-pacted soil and monocropped grass. With the help of community members, she was working to restore soil health and nurture diverse ecosystems for the garden to thrive.

> But [learners from the community are] excited to be out there and people spend time out there, which is really, really cool. I'm going from a pretty much blank space, a defunct bowling green that was just mowed weekly. I know people spend time here in the evenings because I find their beer cans the next morning, but it's been treated perfectly. Nobody's stealing anything. There's no damage, no theft. If anything, the presence of people in here, I think it's protecting the garden. (Barnes 2020)

Community members who work in the garden develop new skills and new rela-tionships. They share knowledge and connect with each other in a space of peace and tranquility—a space safe from the stresses of the outside world. Gardening for food production is hard work. Learning new skills from each other is key, as is learning by trial and error, as Barnes has done, and developing relationships with people one might not otherwise encounter is part of the value of garden education.

Bringing Indigenous Agricultural Knowledge to Farm-to-School and Garden Education Programs

Environmental and agricultural education are key drivers to restoring a just and sustainable food system in any region of the world, even though access to these agricultural education opportunities has drastically declined in recent decades.

The impact of the lack of agricultural education opportunities is all the more pronounced in island nations and spaces due to our closed ecosystems and limited resources. Oceania has a long tradition of passing down knowledge from generation to generation through oral storytelling and experiential learning. These Indigenous traditions were largely erased during colonization and have continued to wane in the larger context of neocolonialism and the global capitalist system. However, in the last decade, there has been a resurgence of interest in Indigenous agricultural and traditional ecological knowledge in both Hawai'i and Aotearoa New Zealand. This knowledge is passed down differently in different places: in Hawai'i, nonprofit organizations promote it in tandem with the Department of Education, however reluctantly on the part of the latter; in Aotearoa New Zealand, this knowledge is disseminated through the marae and the Hua Parakore Indigenous organic certification system and culturally appropriate Māori food production. Although they are not the only mechanisms broadcasting this information, they are among the most successful. Frequently, they are spearheaded or maintained by women.

These different educational contexts reflect the values assigned in each space to Kanaka Maoli and Māori knowledge, respectively. The focus on marae as spaces of knowledge creation and sharing shows a definite emphasis on Māori cultural values. Indeed, many of the Hua Parakore organic food production certification and education programs use the marae as sites of instruction, like Papatūānuku Kōkiri Marae, for example. Conversely, the lack of attention paid to Native Hawaiian agricultural practices is instructive. Even the most well-intentioned school garden programs in Hawai'i focus mostly on western concepts of sustainable agriculture, and seldom include Indigenous food production practices. Native Hawaiian history is included in the fourth-grade curriculum across the state, and Hawai'i schoolchildren plant 'uala (sweet potato) and kalo, and learn about the ahupua'a but that is often the only connection to Native Hawaiian agricultural practices in K–12 or higher education. Colonization's effects are still ongoing, and decolonizing processes have simply not reached enough institutions to be replicated on a larger scale in educational organizations. The case is the same for social justice aspects of agriculture and environmental education. Although there is some focus on Indigenous agricultural knowledge in Aotearoa New Zealand, it is not widespread and is not necessarily included in the formal education that reaches K–12 students. There is even less emphasis on it in Hawai'i and this absence reproduces the current food system's inequalities of access, contributing to environmental and food injustices in Kanaka Maoli, Māori, and other marginalized communities.

At one time, public K–12 schools in Hawai'i had a formal requirement for environmental education, but it was dropped in 1999. The Ka Hei program reinstated a focus on sustainability, but it is geared toward energy efficiency in schools (Ka Hei 2014) rather than involving students in garden projects. Some individual schools value sustainability education, but many do not. The fact that there is no overarching requirement means that education policy has not yet caught up with reality in this era of climate crisis. Given what we learned during the pandemic about the importance of local food resilience in our food system, it would behoove us to educate children to both value local food and to grow it by promoting agriculture as a valid profession. Many school administrators in Hawai'i are descendants of former plantation workers, and all their parents wanted them to do was to get *off* the plantation and improve their lives. The plantation system is predicated on exploited labor, which is what tends to be associated with agriculture. Because land-use policy still favors large landownership, we must devise a new model of agriculture that sustains the population, the land, and the soil. We cannot do that if environmental education is completely missing from the educational landscape.

While Hawai'i may be behind other states in school garden and farm-to-school education, there are many people—again, mostly women—working to catch up and design a culturally appropriate curriculum that values and emphasizes the Kanaka Maoli values of mālama 'āina. Many of these programs are not attempting to reinvent the wheel and take some of their elements from successful programs on the continent. However, they must clearly be aligned not only with State Department of Education standards, but Native Hawaiian culture as well, especially because restoring ancestral abundance is an integral part of the culture.

Several of the respondents shared how they came to understand the relationship between education and sustainable agriculture. For example, Lydi Morgan-Bernal, the statewide coordinator of the Farm-to-School and School Garden Hui, shared that there are multiple ways to approach garden and agriculture education. She approaches it through teacher education programs, as does Summer Maunakea, who explained that the outcomes of 'āina-based education are rooted in the agency of Kanaka Maoli (Maunakea 2019). Morgan-Bernal took a wider view of educating all teacher education candidates in garden-based education.

> How do you get them to be in the garden and learning how to teach with nature as their teacher? Whether it is science, math, language arts, Hawaiian Studies, whatever it may be. How do we build those skills while they're training to become teachers before they get out and work in the workforce so that they'll have more

garden-based learning happening and just general exposure to agriculture, across the spectrum of learning? We are moving forward with that. That's one effort and the Hui has amazing volunteers and I'm the only staff person. But we do have five island networks that really form the framework of who we are. It's all about being in communication with schools and that's the role the island network plays. (Morgan-Bernal 2020)

Morgan-Bernal guides teacher education programs through the School Garden Hui, a network of like-minded education practitioners who develop educational programs in Hawai'i's schools that foster student learning in the garden and educate teacher candidates about including 'āina-based learning in standards-based lessons. Her work is echoed by Lehn Huff on Maui, who retired from teaching in 2008, but was so concerned with the lack of sustainable agriculture education that she went back to work toward this goal. She explained that "what we needed in our islands was a program of returning our students to the 'āina desperately, over every reason imaginable. We can't sustain ourselves with importing food from twenty-five hundred miles away. So that's a no brainer. I think some of us are realizing that now" (Huff 2019).

Many of the women interviewed for this book who work in education focus on K–6 education. In Hawai'i, many middle and high schools no longer provide any avenues for agricultural education and most nonprofits in this sector focus on younger grades to teach children about good food, nutrition, and sustainable agriculture from the youngest age possible. Betsy Cole, while working for the Kohala Center on Hawai'i Island, worked to start a farmer training program beyond high school because she and her colleagues were aware that the university system had a different take on the kind of agriculture they wanted to support (Cole 2019). The College of Tropical Agriculture and Human Resources at UH Mānoa largely perpetuates the current model of industrialized agriculture and focuses on research in biotechnology and other agricultural technologies to improve agricultural output. This educates researchers but does not necessarily educate future farmers. The GoFarm program, also affiliated with the university, has filled some of that void, but it is not graduating nearly enough farmers to make Hawai'i even marginally more self-sufficient. The bias is still that there is little overlap between health and sustainable agriculture.

Prioritizing agricultural and nutrition education is a mission for many of the nonprofit organizations where many of the respondents work. Kōkua Hawai'i Foundation, for example, supports environmental education through experiential learning for Hawai'i's schoolchildren. They "believe our keiki are the seeds of change to preserving and protecting our beautiful islands" (Kōkua Hawaiʻi Foundation 2022). They embrace a collaborative model, engaging an often difficult and recalcitrant partner in the Hawaiʻi State Department of Education to provide garden and nutrition education in schools, align their curriculum with the DOE standards, and improve the quality of food and snacks in public schools throughout the islands. Their work has not been easy, nor has it always been successful, and they sometimes encounter long-entrenched negative attitudes and policies toward school food and school gardens by DOE faculty, staff, administrators, and policymakers. In this antagonistic environment, the Kōkua Hawaiʻi Foundation staff advocated for changes to policies that prevented school garden food from entering cafeterias due to non-competition clauses in the USDA contracts with the DOE. After many years, they were successful in working with other organizations to convince the DOE to overturn these outdated policies.

Kōkua Hawaiʻi Foundation is part of a larger umbrella network of organizations housed under the Hawaiʻi Public Health Institute's Hawaiʻi Farm-to-School Hui. This consortium consists of members from all the islands who work to strengthen farm-to-school and school garden programs throughout the island chain. The statewide coordinator, Lydi Morgan-Bernal, explains that Farm-to-School "*is* the food system because it touches on every aspect [of the food system]." She shares her view of women's roles as leaders in this specific part of the alternative food network movement:

> I would say women probably tend to be more collaborative and communicative and having a statewide network is really about those things as well as community. I feel strongly about the fact that we should be living in community more than we do. Maybe the female way of looking at things is less linear, less separate, and more connective and intertwined. But I do find that willingness to be in constant communication. It's not about a person, it's more about the movement. It's more about the work that needs to get done. (Morgan-Bernal 2020)

This echoes previous respondents' views that the work needs to get done, that the status quo has not worked, and that women are the ones who are willing to take on that work because they see it as intrinsic to a future whereby children and communities thrive when they have access to healthy food. Tammy Smith, also known statewide as "Auntie Tammy" (a distinctively Hawaiʻi-based name indicating respect), is the director of food services at a senior living facility in Honolulu and former cafeteria manager for a variety of charter and public schools. She shares that it is important to "stay focused on our people. It is not only about food; it's about building relationships within you from your communities....It needs to be a passion, but I feel built for this. Women are built for this. We have that instinct of caring" (Smith 2020). Although this view can, again, be construed as essentialist because it ascribes a certain "natural instinct" to women, for Auntie Tammy, the people doing the work are women. She is using strategic essentialism to find shared experiences around what she sees as women's roles as mothers or educators, and not necessarily gender, race, or class as identity categories. Of course, these roles are often gendered, raced, or classed, and there is a danger in using strategic essentialism as a crutch to not have to do the work of finding other common ground based on political goals. Is this a theoretical impasse? Does the use of strategic essentialism remain unresolved here? No. Intersectional praxis comes to rescue—doing the work based on shared practices and lived experiences. As we see in Auntie Tammy's narrative, those in her community who are putting their head down and working to feed people according to their kuleana (responsibility) are women. The work is the important part, not necessarily who they are or what gender, race, or class they identify with. Indeed, her work changes lives daily, building relationships in community for us to all thrive together by having a measurable impact on three hundred children every day through healthy and culturally appropriate school lunches. Indeed, she says that when she makes lūʻau bowls, "without this, there is no us. Plenty of aloha in every stew" (Smith 2020). That is the epitome of combining love for food and connection with culture, sharing knowledge, and resistance to the current food system while simultaneously building a more sustainable food system for all.

Of course, environmental education not only comprises sustainability education—it is rooted in a colonial context. As Ipshita Mitra asserts in her analysis of hooks' and Spivak's work,

> [they] aim to demystify the perception of marginality. It becomes a starting point to write (*read* rewrite) new narratives and imagine alternative "*new worlds*." It almost seems as a project toward decolonising the mind with reference to those sections of society that have been pushed to the background, almost annihilated by dominant forces, and treated as mere shadows with no history or future. Through her intervention in this space, hooks reclaims it as a legitimate one. For her, marginality becomes a space of recovery and resurrection. (2021)

In this view, environmental education is marginalized precisely because it is (and was) associated with a history of abundance and sustaining an entire nation and people with the resources at hand. Reclaiming it is up to us and can be accomplished in a variety of ways. For example, Maunakea's educational journey led her to a faculty position at the University of Hawai'i at Mānoa, where she teaches in the College of Education. Her dissertation research examined the role of 'āina-based learning on educational outcomes, rooted in the genealogy of Kanaka Maoli agricultural practices. Indeed, as Maunakea notes:

> Why didn't we learn these things growing up in Hawai'i, of all places, knowing a genealogy and a history of providing for ourselves on an island and sustaining ourselves on kalo and sweet potato and the ocean and all these things? Obviously, this would have been important for us to learn on a small island. I made this connection that maybe the education we had growing up didn't quite prepare us to make these strong food choices. (Maunakea 2019)

Maunakea made the connection between her Kanaka Maoli heritage, the restoration of ancestral abundance, the decolonization of the food system, and education on her own, despite the Hawai'i DOE.

> Everything I wanted to do is about food and gardening and incorporating that into the curriculum, but mainly looking at health, health behaviors, and family and community health. It was my mission to integrate and create food education at the center of education and then bring in all of the language arts and the math as project-based learning before we were calling it project-based learning. It was simultaneously getting to engage in stream restoration, growing of food and ancestral Hawaiian ways to do with kalo varieties, composting, looking at body forms of Haumea, who is supposed to regenerate soil, give life and birth. (Maunakea 2019)

It is her mission now to change those patterns from within the educational system so that pre-service teachers learn to use 'āina-based pedagogy in their curriculum. She requested that the College of Education at UH Mānoa allot her a parcel of land to teach her students how to teach through the garden, using culturally relevant crops and foods.

> I grew in my knowledge of food and the connection of food with people and how specific to your place that connection really is and then looking at the larger

political implications of restoring normal food systems and what that could look like in terms of self-determination. (Maunakea 2019)

Maunakea had to relearn how to grow traditional foods from her kūpuna (elders) and wants to share that knowledge with her students so that they, in turn, will share it throughout the K–12 curriculum. Like Redfeather, she is clear that ʻāina-based education is not limited to math or science, nor only related to environmental education. It applies across the curriculum and adds "vibrancy to our community" (Maunakea 2019).

The school food movement focuses on food justice as well. Through understanding the relationship between school food and food justice, Betsy Cole developed her understanding of the very real problem of food insecurity in Hawaiʻi schools while working at the Kohala Center and, in true leader fashion, started looking for collaborators to solve the problem throughout the archipelago (Cole 2019). She stated that

> We saw the opportunity in school food that's related to school justice. And I got educated about what was going on with school food and possibly what the business case was for trying to get the schools to buy more food so that our farmers could forward contract and get financing. I know school food is also related to food justice. We have all these kids who aren't getting enough food. They don't eat the school food either. How can we do something about that? Is that going to stimulate the agricultural economy if we can do it right? But mostly, I said, "OK, here's an issue. Let's see what we can do to take it on." And then I looked for collaborators. (Cole 2019)

Not only does Cole's work tie school food justice for children with increasing value for farmers, but she partners with other organizations to increase production and consumption at the institutional level, creating a win-win situation for everyone.

Decolonizing our view of agriculture as exploitative is critical to fixing our food system. We are at a crossroads now, with an opportunity to reshape the policy that dictates what kind of agriculture we support. It is not simply a matter of policy, of course. Assuming that the state will "fix" anything assumes a certain privilege and comes from a view that the state is, at the very least, neutral, if not actually helpful. People who have been colonized, had their land stolen, and who continue to be oppressed by the state certainly do not view the state in this way. Indeed, turning to government to solve problems can have negative effects. Turning to our networks may be more likely to foster solutions. This is not to assert a binary opposition: either the state helps to fix the food system, or our communities of networks do. Rather, it might be more useful to think of the issue as a cluster concept—a both/and proposition. Advocating for the state to reshape education policy and land-use zoning regulations is key, but so too is working both within the educational system (training new teachers in the importance of local food and ʻāina-based practices) and outside of it (gathering networks of like-minded educators and leaders to reshape our environmental education system). These are tactical interventions, with distinct, focused strategies for fixing the food system.

General Agricultural Education

The lack of emphasis and investment in farmer training and education presents serious obstacles to increased agricultural production in Hawaiʻi. Several state programs are in place: GoFarm Hawaiʻi is funded by federal dollars and administered through the University of Hawaiʻi at Mānoa's College of Tropical Agriculture and Human Resources. The University of Hawaiʻi West Oʻahu's Sustainable Community Food Systems is more focused on graduating food system professionals than farmers; it started with funding from Kamehameha Schools and now operates through general funding from the Hawaiʻi State Legislature. However, even combined, they do not constitute nearly the critical mass of farmer training needed to support food sovereignty and increase food system independence in Hawaiʻi. MAʻO Organic Farms is a leader in the private sector in this regard; it trains youth from the Leeward Coast of Oʻahu in significant numbers while simultaneously paying for their education at nearby Leeward Community College and providing them with stipends and opportunities for advancement in the organization. Barnes and Bendixsen found that African American men and women may be unwilling to enter agriculture as a profession due to the generational trauma of slavery (2017). A majority of the population in Hawaiʻi are descendants of plantation laborers, and the idea of young people entering the field (both literally and figuratively) of agriculture is anathema to many parents and grandparents who worked very hard to move off the plantations before they closed in the mid-1990s. In this light, reframing the issue is necessary: both slavery and plantation labor were essentially about dependence and oppression, among many other nefarious outcomes, whereas the goal of food sovereignty is independence and self-determination.

The neocolonial context not only makes it difficult for young people to become farmers due to entrenched attitudes against agricultural work, but it also complicates individual choices to enter farm work or other food system professions. For instance, young farmers working at MAʻO Farms in Waiʻanae, Oʻahu live on a seventeen mile stretch of coast with only two small supermarkets but eleven fast-food restaurants and seven convenience stores. As Jacob (2010) found, "choice" surrounding what to eat, especially in the context of AFNs, is limited when one is marginalized and presented with limited options. Many supposed responses to food system change place the onus on individuals to make appropriate and healthy food choices. However, that notion is "complicated within a neo-colonial context" (Jacob 2010, 366) because the focus on individual behavior places all the responsibility on consumers within a global capitalist framework and relieves the state of any responsibility to support the creation of AFNs, the goal of which would enable greater access to wholesome and fair foods for a larger segment of the population. If the young MAʻO Farms staff has limited access to fresh foods beyond the farm gates, the general population in the area has even less. Neff et al. (2009) argued that this focus on individual behavior is ineffective and can also result in blaming victims for health disparities, environmental injustices, and other inequalities between privileged and underprivileged communities. To address these inequalities, AFN actors must look to Indigenous approaches to food system and agroecological practices.

Cultivating social and environmental change through educational means is one of the undercurrents found in many of the narratives. Sustainability is not a simple premise, especially if it includes social change with regard to living wages for farmers and other food system actors. For example, Emily King's organization is called Spira NZ. The organization's entire focus is to cultivate change by doing advocacy work, running workshops, and training people in food system solutions at both the practical and policy levels (King 2020). Sarah Smuts-Kennedy also envisions training people "on the ground" as her mission. She is trying to scale up her work with communities to create safe bee habitats. She says her task is to be "convincing more than anything. Teaching people on the ground makes you create a movement that can be scaled out and up" (Smuts-Kennedy 2020). These complementary visions focus on different aspects of the food system, yet both women see the value in sharing their knowledge with others and fostering others' growth in order to amplify their respective missions. Jacqui Forbes of Xtreme Zero Waste in Raglan/Whāingaroa, Aotearoa New Zealand explains that agricultural education includes both behavioral change and social change, especially "not throwing things away and revaluing practices of our grandparents such as repair, and reuse, and repurpose, upcycle, those kinds of principles. Now we are just using it once and then throwing it away" (Forbes 2020). Sharing this ethic of care for the land, in this case through waste reduction, is central to changing our conception of what it means to live sustainably. This is larger than "just" agriculture education, to be sure, but it is an inherent component of sustainable agriculture; if people are not educated about their waste, they are bound to continue to consume in amounts the Earth simply cannot accommodate. Waste reduction and understanding one's connection to sustainable agriculture impacts everyone, of course, but as Ness Lotz-Keegan says:

> Educating women in this kind of agriculture is extremely powerful because you're basically killing two birds with one stone. Not only is it education, but it's also food security, and health as well. So it's three birds then. And healthy food for their families. I think food security is going to be a big issue in our developed world. Food and water security for sure. (Lotz-Keegan 2020)

Focusing on women's roles as students and teachers is central to knowledge dissemination. As Lotz-Keegan suggests in her narrative, and as de Schutter (2013) has proposed, women are likely to implement sustainable practices in their own lives and are also likely to impact the way their families consume as well. Although we may decry that it is mostly women who do the time-consuming and tedious labor of shopping for food, that means they have purchasing power. And although focusing exclusively on food spending dollars as a metric is problematic in that it potentially assigns blame or conversely, agency to individuals for their behavior, in the context of daily practices of reducing waste or growing or shopping for food, it is also a source of potential political resistance to the current food system.

Marae and Agricultural Education: Hua Parakore

Many dedicated women (and men) are leading the charge throughout Aotearoa New Zealand to use marae land for regenerative agriculture. They use agroecological principles based in the Hua Parakore system to further food sovereignty and encourage Māori self-determination and health. As Kelly Francis explains, "Hua Parakore is the only food verification system run by Indigenous people in the world. They've got six principles which are based on your spiritual connection to the land and to the people rather than anything else" (Francis 2020). Hutchings explains that

> Hua parakore [a Māori system and framework for growing pure products] food growing is not only about the practice of growing *kai* [food], it is also a political

journey of asserting our rangatiratanga [sovereignty and self-determination] as tangata whenua [people of the land]. For many of us, it is a way of resisting globally driven, multinational agriculture and food production that does not look after the wairua [spirit] of the land or the people. (Hutchings 2015, 16)

This certification framework ensures that foods are free from pesticides and added chemicals. It is based on trust, family, and genealogy. Reclaiming the localness of a food's source has additional meaning if it is grown through the *Te Mahi Māra Hua Parakore* system, often on marae land. Francis explains:

Based on my mother and my whakapapa [genealogy] and the way that I work and my promises and values and everything, they accept my promise, and they don't charge to be certified annually. So it means I, Kelly Francis can continue my promises and continue my connection with the whenua. I am providing food to the community. I can continue that and not have to pay this ridiculous amount [for organic certification]. (Francis 2020)

The Indigenous organic certification system is based on trust and bypasses the cumbersome, western system of organic certification, which involves an exceedingly time-consuming amount of paperwork and costs a yearly fee. However, Hua Parakore does entail a forty-week course to ensure that Indigenous and sustainable agricultural practices are followed and maintained. State-sponsored organic certification does not have an educational component.

Hua Parakore was a system created by two of the high order Māori. They were basically people who were annoyed with the food systems that were in play. So they created something else based on spiritual connection. They drew up a 40-week course for it to be taught to people and it was accepted by the state. They took it to the education department, got approved, and started certifying people with credits to be able to confirm and receive diplomas. There are three or four diplomas based on that now. (Francis 2020)

These courses are often taught at marae in different geographic locations throughout Aotearoa New Zealand. Many of the respondents had gone through the coursework or were themselves instructors in the program. And if they had no connection with Hua Parakore, they had at least heard of it and valued its principles. Pounamu Skelton, an instructor in the Hua Parakore system, saw it as a way of institutionalizing learning ancestral wisdom from her elders. She explained:

We followed the six principles that we'd been informed by from the elders
from our research. I guess what that speaks to is the wealth of knowledge that's
available out there. It was such a privilege. We developed this system, and it was
really gonna be for all people because there is this saying in New Zealand "what's
good for Māoridom is good for the whole" because we look at the world view so
holistically. And for me, it really spoke to me, you know, like this is the way our
ancestors had lived there. They were sustainable. They didn't pollute the earth or
the waterways because they knew that that was their relative. And of course, they
didn't ever over farm because they would move with the seasons. (Skelton 2020)

This holistic worldview is governed by Māori culture and the wisdom passed
down through generations. The fact that it became institutionalized and supported by the state gives it additional legitimacy in the eyes of other, perhaps
even Pākehā, political actors. Arguably, it does not need that additional "seal
of approval" from the state, but the fact that it is institutionalized means that
its structure, and even success, is replicable and can be shared and disseminated elsewhere.

In the context of a colonized Aotearoa New Zealand, marae have long
been seen by Pākehā feminists as sexist spaces because men and women
play different roles in ceremonies and the male roles involve speaking, which
western European culture sees as more valuable (Taonui 2020; Irwin 2019;
Smith 1999). However,

it is incorrect to argue that according to traditional tikanga [tradition] Māori,
Māori women do not "speak" on the marae ātea [courtyard or public area in front
of the marae]. Māori women speak on the marae ātea through various forms of
our oral arts, including whaikōrero [formal speeches] in some areas, during the
formal procedures governing, for example, ceremonies of welcome onto the
marae. (Irwin 2019, 79)

White western feminists might see tikanga as silencing women's voices, but for
Māori women, this does not constitute misogynist behavior. Indeed, Pounamu
Skelton told me while laughing, that "men may speak, but women sing, and
anyway we tell them what to say" (Skelton 2020). This is the epitome of a
Māori feminism, also characterized in part as Mana Wahine Māori, a decolonizing Māori feminist lens aimed at enabling Māori women to reclaim their
place in their own lands (Pihama 2019). It addresses the relationality of race
and gender within a colonial context, going beyond those analytic categories

and being "located within…wider relationships as Māori" (Pihama et al. 2019a, v). It links "well-being, culture, economics and social standing into a matrix that takes account of the individual, the collective and the complex interactions between past and present" (Waitere and Johnson 2019, 91). This framework of valuing women's voices and the marae as a space for an "expression of collective identity" (Tuhiwai Smith 2019, 94) emphasizes sharing, nurturing, and building relationships with other members of the marae "family" and with the land on which it sits. This is not to say that everything always goes smoothly. Cathy Tait-Jameson argued that

> traditionally women would get together and talk about the important things and their community and relay their ideas to men. Traditionally, that's the way it worked. I think what's lost a little bit today is that connection between man and woman. It's pretty rare to get a group of men who will actually listen and believe what a group of women have to say, especially in an Indigenous area. (Tait-Jameson 2020)

Gendered spaces can still erase women's ideas and knowledge creation. This is especially true in traditionally masculine industries, like ranching, or, in Tait-Jameson's case, dairying. The women in this study are working to overcome those barriers and challenges, whether they occur in Indigenous or settler colonial spaces. It is important to acknowledge the issue, but as Adrienne Rich said, "the connections between and among women are the most feared, the most problematic, and the most potentially transforming force on the planet" (Rich 1978, 20). And as Abigail Glickman reflects on Rich's essay, "Disloyal to Civilization," Rich also argued for white women to join with women of color to challenge white supremacy if they truly wished to be transformative agents and good allies as intersectional feminists (Glickman 2019). These two calls to action are clearly reflected in the work of the women working to achieve food system transformation.

Indigenous Agricultural Knowledge

Re-learning traditional Indigenous knowledge is the first step in valuing it as the mainstay of any future agricultural and ecological success in growing food sustainably. Betsy Cole, one of the founders of the Kohala Center on Hawai'i Island, explains that in all of their work, "the Indigenous perspective was very important and clearly still alive. We felt like [we] wanted to combine traditional ancestral knowledge with [western] scientific knowledge and that there was something to offer not only within Hawai'i, but possibly the way we approached issues" (Cole 2019). She explains that highlighting the focus on traditional ecological knowledge and the well-developed Kanaka Maoli agricultural sciences would enable the Kohala Center to focus on energy self-reliance and ecosystem health. This connection between land and people is central to Native Hawaiian, Māori, and many other Indigenous cultures, and it is important to recognize and understand it, so that it can be replicated in today's food system. Oddom explains that "we as Indigenous people did it [made the connection between land and people] every single time, every single meal, every time we planted. There is a real difference in the way you can look at food" (Oddom 2019). Traditional ecological knowledge reaffirms the connection between land and people; food isn't just fuel but confirms ancestral knowledge and genealogical capital. Valuing that connection also reaffirms the agency of Kanaka Maoli. Summer Maunakea shares that

> When your hands are turned up, you have a hungry stomach. When your hands are turned down, you have a full stomach. I look at this education as the vessel for the agency of connected communities to grow their own food and to really have ownership and leadership with their education. I took the form of five bundles of knowledge. They are bundles of knowledge that are meant to be reused, refined, and passed on.
>
> These ancestral food systems are on a continuum. In the schools and in community centers, we are growing food and we are feeding our people and we are educating. Looking at it as regenerative community food systems where we have the ancestral structures for our local youth and all the dry land field systems that produce actually more food than the lo'i. (Maunakea 2019)

The assets or strength-based perspective in this passage is the key here: yes, Indigenous peoples all over the world have been oppressed and suffer from a host of health problems, and they lag behind on numerous social indicators. But a strong network of Indigenous and non-Indigenous actors has been working to change the narrative and are using food to restore healthy and balanced food systems for everyone. Maunakea insists on "looking at a strengths-perspective and assets, what do we all bring, and what do we have around us that we can have a relationship with through growing food, through growing medicine, and through healing our community" (2019)? The last part of her statement most clearly synthesize these key themes. We can heal communities by re-localizing and building a resilient food system. Women are doing much of the work in this arena; their voices showcase how the local food movement in Hawai'i and Aotearoa New Zealand fosters systemic changes in how we educate our *keiki* (children) on the importance of understanding where our food comes from. This is not just about individual behavioral changes, but a larger view on how education can shift mindsets to value local food.

This journey to food system transformation rejects the extractive colonial model of natural resource management and industrial agriculture, and instead embraces an Indigenous world view that acknowledges and respects the interconnectedness of all living and non-living things. This is exemplified through *te ao Māori*, or a Māori worldview. Angela Clifford mentioned that she was hopeful that society could get

> closer to a te ao Māori or an Indigenous world view. That holds within it some massive, massive opportunities to better understand our position on the planet. We need to move as fast and quickly as we can down to a more diverse pathway in terms of power, influence, leaders, and land use. We do have the opportunity to push hard now. It's very front of mind for people to try and create better and more resilient systems. (Clifford 2020)

Rangimārie Mules agrees that the traditional land management systems were incredibly rich and diverse. She wonders how we could "revitalize the [Māori] culture and our place to stand for environmental interaction. We need to move quickly toward being a living example for a lot of these concepts. There is too much emphasis put on the theoretical stuff" (Mules 2020). She specifically notes that there is a relationship between people and the environment, through Indigenous cultural values as applied to modern times. This is not only relevant to people of Māori, Kanaka Maoli, or other Indigenous ancestry though, and that's what makes it so promising as an avenue for change: it challenges society to acknowledge and value complex systems-thinking through the "concepts of agency and cultural identity and societal evolution" (Smuts-Kennedy 2020). Hineāmaru Ropati encourages us to ground that knowledge. She says: "food is the currency in Indigenous societies" (Ropati 2020). Without that focus, much of this knowledge is perhaps too esoteric to be of much use to anyone. Ropati told me that researchers are like scouts: we are looking for cracks in the current food system to make positive changes, not just in theory, but in reality. Similarly, as Skelton reminded me when I interviewed her, "we have to concentrate on our Indigenous views on growing food. What are the practices we used to grow food traditionally? Māori people know this stuff, but education allows it to come through. It's in our DNA. It's traditional knowledge" (Skelton 2020). The applicability of these practices, whether Māori or Kanaka Maoli, is what makes them so important. Although clearly the modern world is facing environmental challenges distinct from those of pre-contact Indigenous societies, their focus on sustainability should center the discussion of food system transformation.

In Hawai'i, those who want to improve the food system tend to work within established state and institutional structures to accomplish incremental changes, pushing the boundaries of programs like the USDA school lunch program, accepting SNAP benefits at farmers' markets, working with businesses to accept EBT cards, tailoring existing school curriculum to school gardens, etc. A few programs and instances go beyond established infrastructure, such as the MA'O Farms social enterprise programs, which trains mostly Indigenous youth leaders from the Leeward Coast of O'ahu to become young farmers or food system professionals, or Farm Link Hawai'i, which has revolutionized the CSA system in Hawai'i, especially during and after COVID, by linking producers and consumers through an online user interface. However, these initiatives are not the norm. Even though these programs are recognized by state institutions, there is no single policy or official state recognition to support the adoption of Indigenous agricultural knowledge in established programs. This means that the necessary systemic changes to the food system only occur incrementally. Hawai'i's lack of political will to decolonize existing processes stems from the lack of established examples for decolonizing other spaces and contexts (Aikau and Gonzalez 2019). Engaging with other spaces in Oceania, like Aotearoa New Zealand, for example, has the potential to shepherd Hawai'i into different, perhaps more progressive directions, and to remake and re-regionalize its own food system.

Food Sovereignty as Food Justice

Food sovereignty is the right of people to define their own food systems through their right to healthy and culturally appropriate foods. This concept is heightened within the context of the colonizing presence of the white European settlers in Aotearoa New Zealand and the descendants of the early American missionaries and the illegal overthrow of the monarchy in Hawai'i in 1893. The land dispossession of Native peoples since western contact contributed to their decreased access to culturally appropriate foods. This ongoing process defines food sovereignty and food justice efforts in Hawai'i and Aotearoa as people seek to reclaim their foodways and cuisines. Food sovereignty emphasizes

> centering the needs of people who produce, distribute, and consume food in our food system and policies, as opposed to markets and corporations...Food sovereignty goes beyond ensuring people in a community have enough to eat. It's about giving people in the community the power to provide or grow food on their own land and improve the relationship between food providers and consumers. (San Diego Foundation 2022)

Food sovereignty extends beyond food access or food security in a single community and encompasses a grassroots movement to transform the food system into a more regionalized, local, and humane food system for both producers and consumers, often through political action. In the context of colonized spaces, the extra layer of decolonizing the food system is central to ensuring that the "grassroots" includes the voices of Indigenous and marginalized people. Indeed, Smuts-Kennedy mentioned that "we need to find more opportunities to engage the community in a way that's meaningful for them. It's something we're still working on and need to do better. In the early days [of any project] you have to keep addressing some of those issues like equity and representation" (Smuts-Kennedy 2020). Similarly, Barnes acknowledges her privileged position in a "Pasifika and Māori community as a white girl being paid to do this stuff" (Barnes 2020). This inclusion and attention to privilege is central to the notion of food justice for any organization or project.

Food justice and food sovereignty were built on one another, though food justice is perhaps more focused on individual communities. Food justice is essentially a movement of movements through a component of everyone's daily life—food. It encompasses factors such as ecological health; environmental justice; racial, gender, and economic justice; and immigrant and refugee rights through community building. It also includes elements like joy, beauty, and peace, which everyone deserves access to as well. Jessica Barnes sees her work as creating a relationship between the garden and the community:

> There's a lot of families who are struggling, so if we can create a space that is really beautiful and welcoming and, you know, "please come in, spend time in here," that's what I would love to create in more spaces as well. I just think this can happen all over the place. You just need people who are dedicated to it. This is my

job. I get paid. It should not be volunteer-based. You need to have someone who
is being paid well and acknowledged for their time and their work. (Barnes 2020)

Barnes's focus on helping struggling families by creating beauty in a garden
space for peace and rehabilitation is great. She is cognizant that women often
give their time instead of being fairly compensated. As problematic as the current
capitalist system may be, this work must be recognized within it, because we
tend to only ascribe monetary worth to those things we value. Barnes should be
paid a living wage for her work because food justice involves creating jobs and
expanding access to culturally appropriate and healthy food. Hannah Zwartz
explained that in

> Kāinga Ora, that's the name for Housing New Zealand that provides rental
> housing for those in need; those farms are all women. They're all working single
> parents. And then at the school I'm working with children and all of those teachers
> are women. And maybe it's also because it is not well-paid work and it's not
> high-status work, but women put up with that price structure. But definitely in
> the kitchen, I think there's hardly any men. (Zwartz 2020)

Zwartz's uncertainty about whether low pay and low status occupations are gendered can be framed this way: does this work incur low pay because it is done
by women? Or is the pay low because social services, teaching, and cooking
are traditionally women's work and therefore less valued? She did not appear to
have an answer. Kate Walmsley was also concerned with this issue:

> I guess like women do have naturally more role of a nurturer. And I think we are
> also celebrated for that. So I think while we might have that innate drive, we're
> also encouraged that way by society in general, perhaps more than men. And I think
> women are also more willing to put in voluntary hours or I guess if we're talking
> about the unpaid economy like women have always been. But from my world
> view, anyway, like it's always been women who have been massive contributors
> to the unpaid economy, to the child raising, and cooking and cleaning and just
> like emotional caring for their families and gardening as well. (Walmsley 2020)

Here, Walmsley decries women's unpaid labor and to this end, encourages
Kaicycle to guarantee a livable wage for all of its employees. She argues that
Kaicycle's work is invaluable and pushing Wellington, and in the larger context

Aotearoa New Zealand as a whole, to address climate change through the various avenues she outlines as follows:

> We want to create living wage jobs in this space and regenerative local food systems in the urban areas, because we need those jobs, you know, like we need that security and stability. And we need this to be a long-term shift, not just like a fad. You know, it is actually really critical work because of resilience and climate change, including food security, including biodiversity, including carbon sequestration. (Walmsley 2020)

Yet in what follows, she reverts to the essentializing notion that women are more aware or involved in people's nutritional needs due to their nurturing qualities. For Walmsley, this gendered view of food and eating conveys the relationship between environmental health, education, and people's health.

> I guess also with the food thing like I'm always concerned about people's food like: "have you eaten enough? Did you eat all your meals today or whatever?" I guess that comes back to the nurturing thing. But like being able to provide or play my small part in ensuring healthy food for people. That does feel like a really important part of what I'm in it for. But I guess it's been more of an environmental focus to me. That's how I got into this space. And through that, I've kind of realized how important the social side of it all and how they interlink and how they feedback positively to each other. (Walmsley 2020)

While a living wage, environmental health, and justice, and meeting people's nutritional needs are all clearly important, they are not the only determining factors behind Walmsley's, Zwartz's, and Barnes's choice of work to transform the food system. As Kate Cherrington argues, the "whole global capitalist system runs on 'more.' That's the way everything is measured, because it stimulates the economy, but what about the natural world, you know? This measure we're all focused on is totally arbitrary and ridiculous" (Cherrington 2020). Kay Baxter, the Aoteraora New Zealand seed saver placed this process of wanting "more" into a larger generational context in relation to food. She equated growing food with women's power:

> I just knew that it was a powerless position to be in and I didn't want to be in that position. We were totally dependent on the northern hemisphere for our food security. No one had any idea. We just gave up gardening. The women basically

went to work so they could have washing machines and electric fridges and carpets in three-bedroom houses, big cars, and all that. They didn't realize when they gave away the gardening, they were giving away power over the quality of the food, and all the rest of it. (Baxter 2020)

Once women relinquished the ability to garden and to grow food, she argues, they lost their power. Angela Clifford echoes this argument, placing that move away from gardening and growing food and toward export-driven agriculture in Aotearoa New Zealand:

We import a lot of the staples in areas like grains, beans, more of those things. And it's from a very non-sustainable source, particularly at the moment. There are very long value chains that are under massive pressure, and we import a huge amount of processed food. So what we tend to do is sell ingredients. You know, we sell milk and import mozzarella. Also, what it means is that we sell the best of our stuff to people overseas who can afford it because we can't afford it ourselves. So that means that people who don't have enough money end up eating not good food. (Clifford 2020)

Many of these organizations and projects are trying to reform a food system that privileges exports and contributes to food injustice, albeit through different mechanisms. Even Jenny Lux, whose organic farm was aimed at being sustainable and turning a profit, saw that her small business also had to have educational and social change aims (Lux 2020). Overall, the respondents' narratives share a clear vision that while we are living in a capitalist system, simply existing within it is not enough. Doing meaningful work focused on community, social justice, and playing one's part in food system reform for the benefit of future generations is an important aspect of living a good life.

"Fairness" in food relates to the labor conditions within which farmers and workers toil to bring the food to market, and to the economic policies that favor certain kinds of markets over others. For example, Daniela Spoto (2019) of the Hawai'i Appleseed Center, explained that the "regular capitalist market-based economy" is not a framework within which we can create solutions to food system woes. Striking the balance necessary between supporting the local food movement and maintaining accessibility for people struggling to make ends meet is incredibly difficult. As a long-time food reporter for the *Honolulu Star-Advertiser*, Joleen Oshiro has followed the development of the local food movement in Hawai'i. She explains

It was ridiculous not to be able to feed yourself local food because it was too expensive. For a while, I was writing this stuff thinking this readership is all there is. These people must be reading this, and it's over their head. They were growing their own vegetables at one time, but it all went away. They got used to the industrial stuff. And now we're talking about this again and they're going to go to the market and pay big money for something local when they can't make ends meet. It's a very complicated situation that we're still grappling with. But I do now write with confidence that if you shop at a farmers' market, that it actually is economical to be able to support local at the same time. There's been an evolution there. (Oshiro 2019)

Land-use policies in Hawaiʻi mean that access to land is too expensive for most people looking to start farming. Regenerating the soil on land that has been farmed industrially for decades would require years of soil remediation to make it suitable for diversified farming. Labor costs are high in Hawaiʻi, as is the cost of living. I dabble in orchard crops and once tried to raise organic meat bird chickens on the side with my former spouse. The final cost of one chicken, barely considering our time to process the chickens, would have been upward of US$70 per 4-pound chicken to account for the organic feed and the chicken tractor materials we bought. This is clearly unattainable for consumers and undesirable for producers. Hawaiʻi farmers and ranchers have made vast improvements in efficiency and there is a high market demand for local products, yet many farmers still struggle to meet consumer demand for their local products. The costs are still relatively high, making local food somewhat inaccessible to people with less money. Improvements to SNAP and its integration into farmers' markets and some CSAs through the Double Bux program have increased access to healthy local food for larger swaths of the population, yet it is still difficult to beat the prices available at big box retailers working within economies of scale. The social justice aspects of AFNs occur in many spaces and through a variety of institutions like businesses, prisons, hospitals, public housing, and perhaps most importantly for future generations, schools.

Networks of Knowledge

School gardens, school lunches, and participation in community gardens are excellent examples of the value of alternative forms of knowledge. Communities of practice and networks of educators are instrumental in the relationship between good food and public health. Tina Tamai, who, as the leader of the Good

Food Alliance, calls herself an "organizer of a network of networks," explains how educating communities about ingredients and nutrition can help improve diet-related disease outcomes.

> If you work with people on a one-to-one level of care, especially with Micronesian populations—no industry group is acculturated to that culture—they are able to come up with ideas. They did recipe cards that were totally pictorial without using words. Then they started to engage people to come to the clinic, and they would have these cooking activities to engage people. But of course, people have different ideas, like "are you really changing behavior by doing that?" (Tamai 2019)

Tamai's concern about the impact of individual behavior change on the food system is well-placed. But there is no doubt on the impact of that individual behavior change when it comes to improved family health outcomes, especially for marginalized communities like Micronesians living in Hawai'i. Her group's educational outreach efforts engage people who may not be able to speak English, or read for that matter, through easy-to-follow illustrated recipe cards for use with locally grown and culturally appropriate ingredients.

> We had fresh fruits and vegetables, so we wanted to promote healthy eating in low-income populations all over the islands, and now it's expanded. The whole idea of using a network of networks is that it is community-based, and that community has a voice, and they determine what their food system should look like. We're trying to support communities who are doing that because we feel like they're the ones that know best. They know what their resources are, so that's why we feel like it should be based on the community's place-based food systems, and then we had the whole idea of gathering all these mini-networks and getting food data to get us to create one big network so that they're intersecting. (Tamai 2019)

The network of networks relied on grassroots input to determine what food sovereignty might look like for each different community. The culturally appropriate foods listed on the recipe cards were requested by community members, who sought access to familiar foods from their home islands.

> I liked my structure, and we decided that really what we were was a coalition of key leaders who were connecting farms and creating distribution systems. So those are the people we kept in the alliance, and we had to ask people to sign up.

It involved economic development too. Let's fix what's broken now. If we don't invest now in these broken food systems, we're going to have [health] problems later. (Tamai 2019)

Tamai's leadership in the Good Food Alliance reflects women's leadership as well as diversity in perspectives, community input, and collaboration, all of which Tamai says are key for success. The nine-member Board of Directors is composed of eight women and one man, seven of whom are women of color. Out of sixteen team participants in the alliance, only two are men, the rest are women—eleven of whom are women of color (https://hawaiigoodfoodalliance. org/about/2022). This organization is building relationships, educating others, and privileging intersectionality to change the food system.

Fostering these connections is central to changing systems. Mules argues that humans are part of systems, and to change the systems, we need to humanize those systems (2020), not maintain them solely on economic terms. Like Tamai, Jenny Lux thinks women have a special role in connecting groups since women are "naturally good social movers and have that community concern. I don't know if we have more of a nurturing role or if we can claim more credit for changing the food system than men, but certainly I connect well with anyone who's wanting to change things" (Lux 2020). Whether these connections are based in a specific culture, the connection of shared food-growing practices and/or skills through gardening, or gendered notions of feeding community, the decolonizing practice of valuing the relationship between humans and the Earth as more than just a one-way resource extractive relationship is key to supporting social justice outcomes. Kelly Francis joked with me that she spent too much time building fancy garden boxes for people when really, for her Whenua Warrior program to take hold and really teach people how to garden and grow food for themselves, she should have spent more time on the relationships and the people (Francis 2020). Although statistics and the number of garden boxes built is a potential marker of success, involving people in the process and increasing time spent with people talking about what they actually eat means that the second round of garden boxes built for folks in marginalized communities was much more successful. Like Smuts-Kennedy's process of co-creating art installations for bee habitats with community, inviting people to imagine a food system revolution with each other is an act of political resistance in and of itself. Women using their voices nourishes community in food justice and sovereignty spaces.

Conclusion

Agricultural education options in Hawai'i and Aotearoa New Zealand have waned in the past few generations. There are some highlights in terms of farm-to-school education, 'āina-based education whether through schools in Hawai'i or through the marae and/or Hua Parakore system in Aotearoa New Zealand. Although they are reaching some students, especially in Hawai'i at the K-6 primary school grade levels, children's exposure to these agricultural education programs decreases as they grow since there are youth and college level programs, but fewer agricultural education opportunities for grades 7-12 (GoFarm Hawai'i 2025). In the United States, some rural areas still maintain 4-H clubs for example, and there has been a small resurgence of interest in these activities. For the most part, however, there are very few agricultural education programs in secondary or post-secondary schools that focus on sustainable practices in farmer training or that formally acknowledge the value of Indigenous agricultural knowledge.

Without the sustainable agriculture educational programs discussed in this chapter—like farm-to-school lunch programs, school gardens linked with curriculum, natural resource academies, Hua Parakore, or even the Sustainable Community Food Systems' concentration at the University of Hawai'i West O'ahu—the current food system cannot be replaced by a more justice-focused food system and food sovereignty cannot be achieved. A food system where self-determination enables citizens to purchase healthy, locally grown food at a reasonable price at the same time as it enables farmers to make a living wage is only possible if everyone understands how it all works. Narratives about "raising awareness" are common but not adequate. It's not enough to educate children about growing food if we do not educate them about fair labor practices, how colonization uprooted Native populations and dispossessed them of their land, or even how Indigenous agricultural knowledge was able to feed millions of people living within finite, island ecosystems with no external inputs.

Agricultural education must be placed in a larger food system context. Understanding how these systems work together is key to achieving a just and sustainable food system within the next generation. Teaching food justice to children and their families through schools, community gardens, marae, waste-reduction facilities, health clinics, and other spaces will transform the food system. The networks of women doing that work now are focused on achieving these goals. Their relationships help to disseminate information and make connections among various food system actors to continue the journey toward food justice and food sovereignty.

CHAPTER 4

Food Sovereignty, Public Health, and Community Nutrition

Eating is an agricultural act.
—Wendell Berry (2009)

School Lunch

The relationship between food sovereignty, public health, and community nutrition actually encompasses diverse areas of the food system. It is inextricably linked with land dispossession, decolonization, and social justice. This work is not a form of activism that one can pick up and leave off. Rather, it is part of a larger system. Food system work and advocacy in settler colonial spaces is a tribute to the generations of Native peoples who came before us and whose illegally occupied land we inhabit. Food sovereignty extends this kind of work. Intersectional praxis encourages us to examine the myriad ways we can fix our food system so that it enables us to feed people good, culturally appropriate foods to increase health outcomes through better community nutrition. These improvements are linked to environmental justice and sustainable agricultural practices because they empower local communities to produce their own food, and they re-regionalize the food system instead of relying on imported industrialized foods or growing food for export. Nowhere are these connections more apparent than in school lunch programs.

The public school food system in Hawai'i is hampered by the kind of cafeteria that most schools rely on. School food services were centralized as a cost-cutting measure starting in the late 1980s and early 1990s, as the sugar plantations were closing throughout the archipelago. Food is cooked in one "cooking kitchen," usually at an area high school, and then trucked and reheated to surrounding "feeder" schools. This structure creates an overwhelming reliance on foods that can easily be reheated and/or that come from pre-made industrial processed foods. It is based on a five-week cycle menu that repeats throughout the academic year. As a parent of two children who attended Hawai'i public schools from kindergarten through high school graduation, I can attest that the menu is heavily laden with processed foods, fats, and salts. For example, the November 2022 menu included pizzas, burgers, sloppy joes, frozen chicken patties, grilled cheese sandwiches, meatball pasta—and roast pork and hot turkey with gravy to mark the Thanksgiving holiday. Chocolate or plain milk, a bread roll, fruit (often fruit salad from a can, but sometimes imported apple or orange slices), and coleslaw or veggie sticks round out the menu. Auntie Tammy Smith, one of the leading experts in culturally appropriate cafeteria scratch cooking in Hawai'i, explains how cafeterias operate:

> Cooking chicken patties makes the most money. Oh, man, that's a multi-billion-dollar industry. Because school kids love chicken patties. That's the number one seller and it has the highest profit margin rate. So how do you stop eating them and how do you compete against that? But we grew up like that. There was fresh food then, but you get plastic today. You [have] no more dishes anymore. We just toss it. Just toss it. You know, like the slop man. We knew he was coming for feed the pigs and it was all good. (Smith 2020)

This model also means that cafeteria staff have lost scratch cooking skills. Cafeteria staff and School Food Services administration staff express ambivalence toward scratch cooking because it adds work for the staff, who are mostly women. Growing food for cafeteria consumption on campus also problematizes the school food chain, whereby most of the food served for school breakfast and lunch comes packaged and pre-cooked. This is another demonstration of the loss of appreciation for culturally appropriate foods. Much of the cafeteria and School Food Services staff are descendants of plantation laborers and replicate plantation food, rather than respecting Indigenous foods. Plantation diets were based on cheap meat like Spam or Vienna sausages, and few vegetables because that is all they could afford. School food is no different and reflects Hawai'i's plantation past.

As Linda Alvarez states regarding food and colonization in Latin America on the Food Empowerment Project website:

> Colonization is a violent process that fundamentally alters the ways of life of the colonized. Food has always been a fundamental tool in the process of colonization. Through food, social and cultural norms are conveyed, and also violated....We must never forget that the practice of colonization has always been a contested

matter as groups have negotiated spaces within this process....Understanding the history of food and eating practices in different contexts can help us understand that the practice of eating is inherently complex. Food choices are influenced and constrained by cultural values and are an important part of the construction and maintenance of social identity. In that sense, food has never merely been about the simple act of pleasurable consumption—food is history, it is culturally transmitted, it is identity. Food is power. (Alvarez 2022)

If food is indeed power, growing and consuming culturally appropriate foods reflects that power and political resistance to colonizing processes. Teaching children to grow their own food, how to cook it, and how to consume the fruits (or vegetables, or meats) of their labor will contribute to fixing Hawai'i's and Aotearoa New Zealand's broken food systems.

Feeding schoolchildren entails a high degree of creativity, patience, and drive. As the cafeteria manager in the central kitchen responsible for feeding multiple schools, Tammy Smith created an entire menu for a charter school on the East side of the island of O'ahu that was culturally connected yet met all the strict federal requirements. She explained that while she was aiming for a 100% Hawaiian focus, she was currently at 75% (Smith 2020). She maintained that it was important to "stay focused on our people. It's not only about food. It's about building relationships within you, from your communities" (Smith 2020). But the federal requirements ignore culturally appropriate foods for Kanaka Maoli. She explained that Native Americans have been able to push federal school lunch guidelines to include beans and greens because they have cultural significance to them. Her discussion underscores the lack of federal recognition of Native Hawaiians:

Beans mean the world to them. Greens mean a lot. And they have all this cultural significance to the Native Americans, but we have none. The government tells us that we need to have a change in our menu. Beans once a week. I mean 'cause, no more connection to beans for Hawaiians, for local people. Not for us. How do we make them understand that? We don't understand beans. (Smith 2020)

She does not begrudge the Native Americans' successful drive to include beans as a culturally appropriate food in USDA school lunch requirements. Instead, she wants Hawai'i to follow suit to push government regulatory agencies to include culturally appropriate foods for Kanaka Maoli, like kalo, 'ulu, and 'uala.

I'll take over the whole school lunch program in the state of Hawai'i. Let me
manage the differences. Changes in people's attitudes about food and how you
care about it because I get it, can just be a job for some, but it also needs to be a
passion. Because no matter what else you feel, food service always is your own
job. Unfortunately, it's looked down upon though. You know, it's a minimum
wage job. But without a change in people's perspective about food service, it's
gonna continue to be an issue. But I feel built for this. Women are built for this.
We have that instinct of caring. (Smith 2020)

Ku'ulei Samson shares Smith's drive to fix the food system through practical
institutional means, but on a smaller scale. As part of her job as the educational program manager at Hoa 'Āina O Mākaha, she encourages participants
to grow their own food, knowing that they will soon realize they can't eat it
all and end up sharing their harvest with their family, neighbors, and other
community members. The word kuleana means responsibility, but also means
a small parcel of land. These small parcels were meant to grow food to share
and distribute with others in the surrounding areas. Samson maintains and
values that knowledge and kuleana now. She says:

It's beautiful being able to work with the 'āina, work with people in my community. I literally live down the road. It's great being able to have a space like this in
my community that I'm able to share, share food, share love, share stories, share
knowledge and always that love comes back ten, ten times, a hundred times plus.
To me, farming is attractive. Mālama 'āina is very attractive. I love it because
I see it as my physical workout time, but it's also my meditation time and my
education time and my "learn something" time. And I get so many benefits out
of this one position. (Samson 2020)

Samson argues that the connections she makes while growing and sharing food are
part of her cultural identity, which maintains the gift economy of her kūpuna, and
fosters networks of support and the creation of communities of practice. It is a central
aspect of a political resistance to a capitalist, colonizing system intended to strip
away cultural identity by reducing access to culturally appropriate foods and crops.
Aotearoa New Zealand does not share the same history of school lunch with
Hawai'i. In addressing hungry children, Emily King explained that

we're dealing with actual poverty. We have one in five kids in poverty. We don't
have a school lunch program. We have a few that are popping up. We don't

cook food with kids, so they go to school hungry. And we have a whole lot of social issues around affordability of food. It's not just about production. I mean, obviously, there is cast on production for environmental impacts and then on consumption for where it's broken because people can't afford to eat much. But, you know, it's not a perfect system by any means. (King 2020)

Not that Hawai'i school lunches are anything to praise—unless they are being prepared by someone like Tammy Smith—but at least they are available. During the COVID-19 pandemic, knowing that school food is sometimes the only hot meal children might have access to in a day, the Hawai'i Department of Education used federal funding to provide two hot meals on a drive-through basis at each school while children were learning from home. Aotearoa New Zealand did not put a similar structure in place. It places the burden of feeding poor children on organizations like Francis's Whenua Warrior, which feeds children culturally appropriate foods. Although outreach to large numbers of children in Aotearoa New Zealand is lower, the intention to feed kids healthy food is present, unlike in most of the Hawai'i school lunches.

Hannah Zwartz updated me on pandemic-related efforts during the state of emergency after Aotearoa New Zealand closed its borders. She said that the school garden she managed started off as a project to grow and cook food just for the school kids, but it outgrew its space. So they

built a brand new, off-the-grid kitchen in a container and are using that to cook for school lunches for different local schools three times a week. They also cook for the café here and do a bit of catering and provide meals on wheels, like to the women's refuge. During the state of emergency, we have been cooking 2,000 meals a week for 50 vulnerable families, distributed by a local marae to their social services clients, using a mixture of our own vegetables and large amounts of diverted food rescue. (Zwartz 2020)

To be clear, this is not being done through the schools or any state institution; rather, Urban Kai Farms took on the task of feeding vulnerable families in marginalized communities. Angela Clifford mentioned the lack of state in-volvement as a specific problem that Aotearoa New Zealand needs to address. She argues that

we need a national food strategy, our own food ministry rather than being the marketing department. We are calling for a citizenry of food. An ability to feed ourselves in a self-sufficient and culturally appropriate way through crisis kitchens, because we're looking at really huge food access and food poverty statistics as we move over these next few months [early on in the pandemic]. Activating the redundancy in hospitality to feed people with government and industry support. It's a really big project. (Clifford 2020)

This work embodies decolonizing our diets. Kaui Sana interprets this process as a "basic, basic human right of fairness, and equality" (Sana 2019). Attaining these fundamental rights is inherent in the process of pushing against neocolonialism whether within institutions, like schools, prisons, or hospitals, or outside of them through alternative means. Examining foodways through an intersectional lens is simply one way to understand this process.

Nutrition and Environment Connection

Women tend to be blamed for the obesity epidemic if they work outside the home and do not have time to cook from scratch for their families. Holding women up to an impossible standard of "doing it all" and cooking healthy whole foods for the benefit of our families' health puts women in an untenable situation. Glover et al. (2019) argue that the food provisioning choices of Māori parents and caregivers, who are mostly women, are influenced by cost, price, time, lack of help, fatigue, family members' varied food preferences, and the possibility that children will reject unfamiliar foods. The rise in obesity, and specifically in the obesity rates of Māori families, has been attributed to the combination of these factors. Centering any response to these diet-related health matters around Māori values is critical to successfully remediating them. From a public health and nutrition perspective, Glover et al. (2019) suggest that counteracting the "dependency created by colonization and the associated 'cultural imperialism,' which have prevented Māori capacity to establish culturally relevant *tikanga* (codes) for living that protect against modern threats to health" (13) is key. Field-ing-Singh also argues that families with low socioeconomic status tend to ascribe symbolic meaning to food deprivation (2017), which complicates the story of food within a neocolonial space. She found that food was an important exception to the scarcity that surrounds the daily lives of people living in poverty. Parents can use "food to compensate for other domains of scarcity, thereby emotionally satisfying [children] and bolstering parents' own sense of worth as responsible caregivers" (Fielding-Singh 2017, 425). Although her research centered on adolescents who were old enough to make food requests to their parents in San Francisco, one of the most expensive cities in the world, her findings about the symbolic value of food as an inexpensive way to provide something that a child wants extend to other communities.

In Aotearoa New Zealand, many respondents aimed to combat chronic, diet-related illnesses by providing access, knowledge, and education about food and sustainable agriculture, as well as culturally appropriate foods. Nevertheless, tangible solutions are difficult to discern given the current disconnect between nutritional knowledge and traditional ecological knowledge. For example, Emily King, the director of Spira New Zealand, explains that "dietitians are grappling with what we should do about this. We have never been trained in debilitating diseases or even trained in health issues. How do we take into account the impacts of our recommendations on the environment as well" (King 2020)? Sarah Smuts-Kennedy shares another series of points about this relationship:

> We started to call it urban farming but it's really infrastructure that delivers carbon sequestration, biodiversity well-being, air filtration heat sinks, water retention and harvesting, soil remediation, local resource, organic waste in terms of composting local jobs, all to fight climate change. Food security, nutrition security, because the six-figure farming model actually doesn't deliver nutrition security. Social cohesion and optimism are key. (Smuts-Kennedy 2020)

This list of environmental connections to nutritional needs and food security is also rooted in a broader vision articulated by Jacqui Forbes, the executive director of Xtreme Zero Waste in Raglan/Whāingaroa, Aotearoa New Zealand. She makes the following point:

> We're about health and well-being. So that's a broader vision in which we move, working in space to achieve change, health, and well-being. Because for us [Māori], our diets are really bad. Assets are like the nutrients in the soil, the nutrients in the plants, too. And for our bodies, you know, the potential that we don't even really know that exists from eating nutrient rich foods. (Forbes 2020)

Forbes's work in waste reduction fosters connections between nutrients in food and in bodies. She articulated probably one of the most powerful statements of the entire Aotearoa New Zealand research. She told me that she was tired of being at the "bottom of the cliff" and dealing with waste and issues *after* they had happened—like community and public health problems, environmental pollution, and food insecurity. More precisely, she said: "sometimes I think everyone should just move to the top of the cliff and design it out like if we all moved up there and put all the energy up there" (Forbes 2020). She would prefer to focus on prevention, instead of dealing with problems after they arise. Forbes thought that if we put our energy into soil health through regenerative agriculture using proven Indigenous practices, the nutrients in food would necessarily be higher, and people's health would necessarily improve through better nutrition.

To this end, embracing traditional practices within a modern context is a constant challenge. Doing this means stepping into a world where culture and identity are inextricably woven into community and place, as well as another world that is shaped by legislation and policy. For example, Healthy Families New Zealand bills itself as being part of the growing movement to place Indigenous knowledge and practices on an equal level with western epistemologies. This means privileging the views of Māori as principal bearers of our knowledge, rather than as a drain on the health system, or a financial cost for New Zealand to bear (Healthy Families NZ 2023). Furthermore, Vandevijvere et al. (2019) focused on a large study of obesity in Aotearoa New Zealand and found that a large-scale systemic nutritional policy view was important for strengthening accountability of all the major actors within the food system. Theirs was the only study in the academic literature that did not focus on individual behavior change, as it relates to healthy eating, but rather on policies at the international and national levels. The conclusions of this study are a big shift away from placing responsibility on individuals and certain communities to "make the right choices at the supermarket," to use the language of consumption capitalism, and a big shift toward incorporating traditional ecological knowledge into sustainable agriculture practices.

Women and Food

Women have had to become community experts in the food system space. In Hawai'i, Rachel Ladrig said that she was trying to foster connections because she found she did similar work to others through a variety of networking opportunities for grassroots organizers (Ladrig 2019). Kaui Sana, the MA'O Farms manager said that it is "women who emerge as the leaders. It's women asking: how do we take responsibility and think ahead" (Sana 2019)? She characterizes her work at MA'O as being a "strategic attempt to heal community, to give access to fresh food, to families, educate young adults and graduate them with college degrees" (Sana 2019). Indeed, these leaders and organizers can take all kinds of forms and emerge from all different kinds of spaces. For example, Alicia Higa and Moulika Hitchens from the Wa'ianae Coast Comprehensive Health Center (WCCHC) are definitely experts in their community. Higa shared that she saw "all the health disparities related to lifestyle opportunities, not even choices, because sometimes you don't have a choice" (Higa 2019). To address these disparities, she created the WCCHC farmers' market. She explains:

> Our markets are not like regular farmers' markets. We're really food justice markets. We're truly there to provide access. We do have prepared food vendors in, but they're required to follow certain guidelines, provide the healthy options using local agriculture. But we're really there just to provide access to fruits and vegetables, local meat, simple eggs. And the prepared food vendors kind of help pay the higher fees. We were the first farmers' market on the island to take SNAP. (Higa 2019)

At the same time, connections are made to the locally grown products for sale that day, ensuring that the connection between environment, nutrition, and health is front and center.

> We also have a Keiki Prescription Program. We created a program that allows our pediatricians to write prescriptions for fruits and vegetables to the kids that come to our clinics. We just piloted phase one and we're in phase two now. We're gonna get ready to start writing prescriptions from our food distributions because we know that people won't cover it. They're already food insecure and we really want to make sure that we're hitting them when we have access to them so that we're hitting that population. Everybody is creating a component for this prescription program for which we already have secured funding. My goal is to really expand this program and hire more of the kids from West O'ahu because it's needed. They know their community. They're the experts. I want them to come up with the next ideas of what needs to happen. I've been here a long time. I might be out of ideas soon. (Higa 2019)

Working with doctors at the Wai'anae Coast Comprehensive Health Center, Higa and Hitchens promote the preventative medical benefits of healthy food for children and families. The Keiki Prescription Program was included in a feasibility study to measure its long-term impact on health outcomes for participating area residents. Esquivel et al. (2020) found that participants reported lifestyle benefits for children and family members who received the prescription for fruits and vegetables and filled it at the WCCHC's farmers' market. Monica Esquivel, one of the authors of the study and an Assistant Professor and Dietetics Program Director at the University of Hawai'i at Mānoa (UH Mānoa), echoes the importance of this program. She argues that health maintenance organizations like the Hawai'i Medical Service Association (HMSA) and Kaiser Permanente Hawai'i pay for people to go to the gym, "so why aren't they paying for kids to make sure they get fresh fruits and veggies, things like preventative care as opposed to paying for trying to fix the symptoms later" (Esquivel 2019)? The focus on preventing disease through food is nothing new, but systemic barriers in the health care system as well as the current food system prevent us from taking advantage of these opportunities.

The sheer amount of work involved in righting the sinking ship of the broken food system is nothing short of enormous. But women are the ones taking on the task. They tend to be poorly paid and unrecognized for it, but they are persevering. Many of the narratives surrounding food, food access, and healthy and nutritious foods for family and community are based in the notion that women are nurturers. Dr. Matire Harwood, Associate Professor of Māori Health at the University of Auckland and General Practitioner at Papakura Marae Health Clinic, echoes this idea. She says women "have a natural tendency for nurturing. We need to think big. But the [men] love the power, love to be seen making the big decisions" (Harwood 2020). In the next breath, Dr. Harwood's colleague jokingly chimes in to say that in her experience, the work is not paid and that much of it is done on their own initiative. Dr. Harwood jumps in and retorts

> it's kind of a joke having a sense of social justice and wanting to critique the system. We are tired of the patriarchy, so we quit working in it. We have to take a feminist lens to think. It's what drives a lot of our work as well. It's sort of guerilla grassroots. (Hardwood 2020)

The sense of feminist social justice in the public health sector drives these women to continue their work, whether they are supported by large institutions or doing "guerilla grass roots" work on their own to serve their communities. This ethos is rooted in a sense of feminist social justice that adopts nurturing as a path toward transforming public health, instead of viewing it as essentialist or problematic.

The basic act of feeding community and/or feeding families is central to many of the narratives as well. Ness Keegan's discussion of nutrition as medicine demonstrates this concern for family health. Her interest in maintaining the well-being of her family was central to her journey toward cooking healthy meals. Her son "was diagnosed with an autoimmune disease. He lost the use of his limbs and [the family] found their way through it through nutrition and dietary changes" (Keegan 2020). She had always been interested in plants and their medicinal uses, so altering their diet was a way to integrate both aspects of nutrition for health. That connection is also present with the permaculture students at PermaDynamics. Many students are women who come to learn at the PermaDynamics farm because they have experienced health issues, either for themselves or for their families. They want to learn how to have access to healthy food with the shortest supply chain possible to benefit from the most nutrients in the food. Frieda Lotz-Keegan explained that there is a "big connection with nature and nutrition and healing that was traditionally women's role, so it could be an intuitive response to the crisis that we're in. There is a connection between nutrition and health of both ourselves and the land" (Keegan 2020). Yet, do we run the risk once again of relegating women to doing the emotional and physical labor of feeding their family and community food to ensure their ongoing health and well-being? Does this reproduce the gendered, raced, classed, and even colonized focus on women in the kitchen? Does it heap various identities into a pile of intersectional oppression when the entire point of changing the food system is to ensure it works for everyone—no matter their positionality? Hannah Zwartz argues that performing these tasks is just the reality of women's lives, no matter how much we would like to claim that it is not. These realities may, however, be the basis for finding common ground—regardless of race, gender, class, or indigeneity—among women to push for food system transformation. Yes, "women take on more responsibility for food, especially in a traditional household, or most households. This may be an overgeneralization, but probably women are overrepresented at doing unpaid work in the kitchen" (Zwartz 2020). This reflection on the problematic notion of "women's work" is relevant in myriad ways, and not always negatively. Mules said that

> We must balance pragmatism and empathy and compassion in all our interactions, to multi-task. Basically, the human story of female attributes. I'm not saying that men don't have that. But I think women possess these abilities a lot more consistently. I think it helps you be a person of the land and be someone who looks at feeding others and being part of cyclical notions of things. (Mules 2020)

This connects women with food, but at the same time, we can look back to that relationship as one of caring, giving, and, to a certain extent, joy at being part of a larger whole. As Hineāmaru Ropati reminded me, one does not have to be a mother to have what she called "motherly ways. We're natural food harvesters, we multi-task, when we find even our last piece of energy to satisfy everybody around us" (Ropati 2020). Coming up with ideas, planning, shopping for food, or growing food based on a perennial diet, as Lotz-Keegan and Keegan have done (2020), and cooking it are certainly difficult, time-consuming household duties, and more often than not, they are performed by women. Yet they are also a starting point for understanding how the food system works for or against us and for using that knowledge to foster change and build AFNs based on trust.

Indeed, it can even lead to a life's work in various sectors of the food system. Kay Baxter's seed-saving work arose precisely out of a concern for what she was feeding her family, a clear reflection of Spivak's strategic essentialism. She described this journey in the following way:

> I was very naive when I started on this journey specifically as a mum. I cared about what I fed my kids. I've got no science background at all, although I've learned a lot. I also didn't know anything about what happened in this land. I know around the western world, when we wanted to earn export dollars, so we could import to have a higher standard of living, and what that means and the implications for our food. I hadn't understood that. I was staunchly organic right from the beginning. I've always been an organic advocate and practitioner, but I didn't know anything about biological agriculture. (Baxter 2020)

When she first started her seed-saving work, Baxter explains that she had to learn about sustainable growing practices, but also educate herself about the history of land management in Aotearoa New Zealand. She did not mention Māori gardens or agricultural practices directly though, which rankled some of the other interviewees who mentioned this important omission in Baxter's work as problematic.

> The seeds that have actually co-evolved within living soil are the only ones that have got feedback loops with the microbes and the fungi in the soil. And they're the only ones that are able to pick up everything they need from the soil in order to get 90 percent of what they need from the universe. They actually are the only ones that sequester carbon in the process of growing, and build soil, and regenerate. Otherwise, we don't get nutrient dense foods in general. It's about our health and animal health and ecological health. (Baxter 2020)

Through trial and error, Baxter learned the scientific aspects of healthy soil eco-systems and their impact on the nutritional value of foods. This demonstrates the connection between nutritional health and environmental well-being.

> I had to learn the science to support what I'm feeling before I could really talk about it. I now understand that for the human DNA to remain strong and for us to be healthy and for our next generations to be healthy, we have to eat a nutrient dense diet which requires strong genetics and a strong environment. And to grow to grow nutrient dense food, you've got to have the right seeds. (Baxter 2020)

Baxter's role as a mother engaged her to learn more about nutrition to feed her children healthy food. Then she taught herself about organic agriculture, and nutrients in the soil and in the food she was growing, leading her to save seeds selected for nutrient density and overall health of the plants and food she was feeding her family. She also problematized it within the global capitalist system of focusing on exporting food to import goods previously unavailable in Aotearoa New Zealand. As she explained, her kids' health was what started her on this path to learning about her surroundings, the economic system she was a part of, its colonial roots, and how this affected the food available. Interestingly, Baxter did not explicitly mention the land dispossession of Māori, yet she did mention that the western world's perspective on land management combined with public health makes no sense. Instead, she argues for being outside the mainstream so that she can feel good about the work she does. She reflects that while it is important to ascribe a monetary value to her work and her seed-saving practices, it is also an important part of forming AFNs through seed saving from the ground up.

Cultural Identity: Food Is/As Culture

Although Hawai'i is the most isolated populated landmass in the world and is (mistakenly) considered by some to be a "racial paradise," or what Jonathan Okamura has called an expression of multiculturalism at its best (2024)—a melting pot of races and ethnicities where everyone gets along—we have already established that it is in fact a settler colonial space with many associated problems. As Aikau and Gonzalez (2019) explain, Hawai'i has a

reputation as a multicultural paradise adding color to a holiday experience…
While this place is indeed beautiful, it is not an exotic postcard or a tropical
background with happy hosts. People here struggle with the problems brought
about by colonialism, military occupation, tourism, food insecurity, high costs
of living and the effects of a changing climate. (1)

That said, it is also a cultural crossroad, with food at the center. Food is a part
of one's cultural identity on a global scale. Hawaiʻi and Aotearoa New Zealand
are no different. This is another instance where intersectionality is made even
more complex when examining food systems–it shows us how we can move
our understanding of power and social justice through uncovering stories of the
relationship between food and cultural identity, and how food can foster cultural
revitalization. For example, Kaʻiulani Oddom, the Roots Program director at Kōkua
Kalihi Valley, recognizes eating as an act of decolonization—of reclaiming one's
food system, one's culture, one's health—and understands that it supports healthy
communities as well. She explains: "we as Indigenous people did it every single
time, every meal, every time we planted, all of that. There's a real difference in
the way you can look at food. I have the science background, but I also have a
cultural backdrop" (Oddom 2019). She knows that eating culturally appropriate
foods has implications that go beyond individuals. It creates community and
creates spaces for different cultures to thrive. This is intentional. She created
structures and activities at Kōkua Kalihi Valley in order for that to happen. For
instance, Oddom explained:

> We started to collect data and after that we started having dinners over here. I'm
> asking people to tell stories of health and we collected items for four months
> and what we came up with was what we call a *hā* or four connections. And those
> connections took place, connections past and present. But for us, it's culture.
> (Oddom 2019)

Establishing the relationship among people, among cultures, and among Indigenous epistemologies centers Oddom's work. The Pasifika and Native Hawaiian health stories result in rich ground for research and practice to serve the
surrounding community. They also focus on an assets-based perspective—how
do we demonstrate our health practices? How do we determine that culturally
appropriate foods improve our diets?

But in all of the stories that we're told about health, these are the connections people were making. No matter what programs I run, no matter what metrics I have to do, I need to make sure I'm building these connections all of the time, and so we've been using that as a framework. In fact, our staff gets trained on it. This is what we know is important to our community. We base a lot of what we do on these connections. We came with a strong cultural background into the work that we do. And that was important in that we were able to bring cultural components. Almost everything I do has a cultural component. That helps to open the doors into a food system that people may not have come into. (Oddom 2019)

While western grant-making institutions ask for certain metrics like body mass index and other western concepts of "health," Oddom suggests that including Native culture in all of the Kōkua Kalihi Valley health programs is more of an indicator of well-being than body mass index (BMI), rates of diabetes, or heart disease. As Thirkill argues, race is not a determining factor of ill health, but racism is (2021). BMI is a numerical representation of this issue in the public health sector, and Oddom's opposition to its use reflects this pocket of resistance through place-based alternative practices that use culture and food to bring people together. These metrics do have a place in her analysis, but she argues that they are not the only measure of community health.

We would give the staff $50 on a Friday if they wanted to make food from their own ethnic background. At the lunch hour, people would bring handmade things from their culture. They'd do slide shows. They'd dress up in costume. But it was the first effort to make people proud of their food, proud of where they were from, and to tie that all together. Since then, over eight years, we got the community garden too. We have a cultural food hub where we work with 13 organic farmers to bring in food that we sell to the community at a very low market discount. (Oddom 2019)

Encouraging her staff to share their cultural foodways and traditions was another step in connecting with community and patients. And since many of the Micronesian folks who come to the health center in Kalihi have rural and agricultural backgrounds, she learned that they would be only too willing to come to a community garden and grow culturally appropriate crops that reminded them of home.

My work for me is very personal. I was doing all the right things. But I actually ended up taking science in school because what happened in school to us, this was before a lot of the traditional Wai'anae diet programs and all of those things, there was no research really on Native Hawaiians and diet culture. I would end up having to get permission to do interviews instead of being made to look in the library. (Oddom 2019)

Oddom's educational and employment journey exemplifies how Indigenous people have had to both navigate colonized spaces and maintain energy and create space to honor their own traditions. In the grants she applies for as a part of Kōkua Kalihi Valley, she is still asked to use BMI as a metric for success, even though it has been shown to be an irrelevant marker of one's general health. It remains an important data point for grant-making institutions because it is privileged by a white western society, but it essentially reproduces the structural racism of colonizing practices by forcing people to conform to a Eurocentric ideal of a healthy body without considering different body types and shapes. Oddom is working to reclaim language that works against those for whom she advocates, much as Lorde (1984) used the language of transformative feminism to advocate for marginalized peoples. Pounamu Skelton explained that she could see the nutritional deficiencies in her community:

I could see what was going on with the western models of health was failing us. People are really unwell and we're overweight. We've moved to western foods and we're over sugared and we're now gluten intolerant. And all these experts and the estimates are happening in schools, and I wanted to help be part of the movement to move young people toward wellness, which is not just old knowledge, but we needed to find another way to spread the message. (Skelton 2020)

Skelton explained that her work with Hua Parakore was multifaceted. It was not based solely on better nutrition, but also included gardening and reclaiming Māori gardening methods, which all led to an increased sense of well-being. More specifically, she said:

I forced myself to go outside, put my hands in the dirt, didn't do anything in particular, just mucked around with my hands in the soil for 20 minutes. My barometer, my Māori levels, just came right back up to wellness. There is something really healing about working in the soil. Pre-contact we had no synthetics, pesticides, herbicides going onto the land and our ancestors used to use all kinds of tricks to create really healthy food systems and gardens. And then, of course, we used to move around a lot. When the fish were running by the rivers, we would be there collecting food, when the birds were in the bush, we would be there and then we'd have these gardens we'd work for a season. (Skelton 2020)

This discussion of seasonality, sustainability, and only taking what one needs recalls Chapter 2's discussion of land stewardship through Indigenous agricultural practices and connects it to a sense of overall well-being through which to overcome nutritional deficiencies and public health problems like chronic, diet-related diseases.

Indigenous peoples are well-versed in these concepts, even if they do not necessarily name them as such. Their ways of knowing and understanding the world are the very definition of sustainability, and western epistemological views have only recently come around to value them. Kelly Francis, working at Ihumātao Village, explained how her group provided food access to children in the nearby community who were hungry.

And we had a lot of kids who were coming around, who were sick, who were hungry. We noticed a lot of habits and things that could change if we were together. So we built this garden and it was based on the things that we cherish as Māori. Meaning we did one in the shape of a marae, one in the shape of a river, one in the shape of a mountain, and grew staple foods so that the families who would eat from them understood how to harvest and cook. We also did a breakfast club garden which allowed the kids to come in first thing, grab all the food, go in the community to cook it for breakfast and come back round the orchard where they would pick fruits and things and then come back and go to school. (Francis 2020)

Similar to Oddom's work at Kōkua Kalihi Valley, Francis's work to feed hungry and sick children is rooted in Indigenous values and culturally appropriate gardening practices. She claims that the link between Māori culture and healthy food is key to creating and maintaining a relationship between the kids and good food.

It's like the informal food system. If you remove the idea of ownership and all of that kind of thing and glorification and gratitude and all of those things, if you take away all of those expectations and all those levels that you expect to have from somebody, you'll be left with the fact that somebody ate your silver beet [swiss chard] that you grew with your heart and your soul and you put your blood and tears into it and picked and took it down to a woman that has six children. She ate that, she got the nutrients, she got the spiritual connection, she got the love from you. Nothing else matters, you know? (Francis 2020)

The language of what Francis calls the "informal food system" is instructive here. Giving food to neighbors and sharing the abundance of one's garden with friends and family, is a central tenet of Māori-ness. No money is exchanged, and yet it is not bartering. There is no expectation of anything in return. That is a far cry from any western conception of a food system. The gifting and sharing of food were evident in many of the Aotearoa New Zealand narratives, but Francis's inclusion of love really highlighted its importance.

> The reward that you get is the look in your auntie's eye. When you give her the silver beet, that's the reward you get. And that's the reward you expect, and you don't expect any more, or any less because you've already spiritually connected to her so much that it doesn't matter as long as she enjoys the mana that's inside it. There were spiritual ways of connecting to the food system as the only food here, [the] only Indigenous food verification system in the world. And it's one that relies on a promise. We when we feed, we feed mentally, spiritually, and physically. We feed on challenges. (Francis 2020)

Understanding the interdependence of our relationships with the land is rooted in most Indigenous cultures. It is up to the western world to catch up and move toward implementing these concepts on a larger scale to turn back the clock away from the inevitability of climate change and species extinction. Additionally, these practices have the potential to reconnect people with their food. As Huambachano (2019) states, "food rehydrates cultural memories" (4), and it is vital to incorporate food not only as sustenance but also as a powerful symbolic device that connects communities and families, to renew relationships both to each other and to the land.

The availability of culturally appropriate foods in communities illustrates the distribution of power. It is not simply the existence of "good food" or "bad food" in a specific community, but a larger reflection of the agency of that particular community to access culturally appropriate foods through the work of women *within* those communities. They are not outsiders and they have built up credibility over time. Many of the narratives about food deserts and food insecurity, as problematic as they may be, reflect histories of land and cultural appropriation. Monique Fiso, the chef/owner of Hiakai NZ in Wellington, with whom I exchanged emails but did not have a chance to interview due to scheduling conflicts, has successfully reclaimed Māori stories and foodways. *Lonely Planet* and *Time* magazine have both called Hiakai, which means "hungry" in Te Reo Māori, one of the best Indigenous food experiences in the world. Fiso worked for seven years in New York, cooking other people's visions, but returned home to Aotearoa New Zealand in 2016 to revive her ancestral foodways. She researched archival texts to re-discover Māori recipes and ingredients. Her innovative approach reflects her respect for Indigenous ingredients. The Hiakai website describes the restaurant's mission as "challenging the status quo of Māori food in New Zealand, while playing a leading role in keeping Kai Māori and Polynesian food culture alive" (https://www.hiakai.co.nz/about). This Indigenous food revival is not only occurring in Aotearoa New Zealand. For example, chef Sean Sherman of the Oglala Lakota Sioux tribe working in Minnesota prioritizes Native foods and leaves out imported and what he calls "colonial ingredients" to contribute to the decolonization of Native foodways. Sherman explains that "if we can control our food, we can control our future. It's an exciting time to be Indigenous because we can use all of the teachings from our ancestors, and apply them to the modern world. This is an Indigenous evolution and revolution at the same time" (Sherman 2022). Hiakai's cuisine is not aimed at underserved populations, unlike much of the rest of the work described and examined in this chapter, but it does attract national and international attention for Māori cooking methods and re-ascribes value to Indigenous ingredients.

Colonizing practices use food, or the lack thereof, to undermine Indigenous cultural identity. In turn, many communities engage in political resistance by sharing knowledge about food during social gatherings, which leads to community building. Be it a large or small gathering, a formal or informal event taking place in Hawai'i or Aotearoa New Zealand, food is always central to the occasion. For example, it would be unthinkable for a guest to arrive at one's home empty handed, without a special dish to share. On a larger scale, some of the women interviewed for this project made it their life's work to share culturally appropriate foods in a variety of venues and institutions.

Cooking Food, Growing Health

The relationship between good food and good health is clear in both the medical and social sciences literatures (Centers for Disease Control 2023; World Health Organization 2023; Wahl et al. 2017; Harvard School of Public Health 2017). Building on this book's earlier call for focusing on an assets-based perspective of Hawai'i's and Aotearoa New Zealand's food systems and their relationship to health, this section identifies how participants viewed cooking as integral to a sustainable food system as well as a contribution to the health and well-being of residents in both locations. In finding good quality, local products for cooking, Sarah Burchard extols the virtues of farmers' markets for residents and visitors alike. She leads a Kakaʻako farmers' market tour on Oʻahu to highlight local and seasonal ingredients. She has also

> hosted farm-to-table events in the past called "Pupus [appetizers] with a Purpose." I bring in a farmer or rancher and they do a talk throughout the meal, and I cook with their ingredients. Everything I do is to support local. Most of the restaurants that I support, support local farms. I hope to bring a little bit of education and encourage people to not only start supporting local, but also for them to encourage others as well, as a kind of ripple effect. (Burchard 2019)

Burchard's goal is to feed people good food and educate them at the same time about the difference between Native Hawaiian cuisine and local cuisine, to include some history of foodways in Hawaiʻi, and to highlight the things people can do to support an alternative food system that values small producers and local farms. She explains, for example, "I did a project in 2018 called 'The Year of Ingredients' on Instagram (@yearofingredients), you'll see that every single day I posted a different local ingredient, what it is, and how to cook with it" (Burchard 2019). Burchard uses social media to spread messages about the importance of local food to various communities. She purposefully reaches out to young people to encourage them to seek out local ingredients. Learning how to cook with them is a key component of reaching different demographics and people who might not otherwise have access or awareness about the importance of food system transformation.

> So there's a little bit of education about what the local ingredients are, where to get them and how to cook with them. It encourages people to cook with them and also inspires them. But then with our dinners and certainly with the farmers' market, it's half about exposing people to ingredients and enticing them to eat them and half about explaining to people why it is so important, how it's good for our economy, how it's good for the environment, how it's good for food security, how it connects you with the land and connects you to your community. Those are all the things that I try to touch on with a lot of my work and then with my food writing too. I profile a lot of local food entrepreneurs. A lot of times the restaurants that I write about are using local ingredients as well. And I give a shout out to the ingredients they're using, trying to put it out there as much as possible so people get used to hearing it. I feel like the more you hear something, the more you are going to want to do it. (Burchard 2019)

As a chef, she cooks with local ingredients to support and highlight the environ-mental and health benefits of local food. Admittedly, her clients tend to be from a higher socioeconomic status. In contrast, Monica Esquivel's work as a former health promotion director at the Waiʻanae Coast Comprehensive Health Center and now a professor of nutrition and dietetics at UH Mānoa focuses on reaching out to underserved communities in innovative ways in order to reach them where they are. For example, one of her grant projects with the USDA was to

> train more Native Hawaiian, Pacific Islander, Filipino dietitians [because] one argument is that it reflects the people they see, but they also reflect the culture. They are the ones that can make sure that these recipes for the schools and the menus for the school are culturally appropriate instead of the beef stew that's supposed to be from plantation days. (Esquivel 2019)

Jessica Barnes argues that cooking seasonally is cheaper and of course better for the planet. Her work on low-budget cooking literacy focuses on doing small cooking workshops because she sees "a need in the community around a lack of literacy around cooking healthy food on a budget" (Barnes 2020). Indeed, Cherrington explains that budget cooking is related to conceptions of wealth as well. She laughed when she said:

> a real strange thing is that people really measure wealth in the western world by having a lawn. You know, the measure of wealth is the length of your lawn, and your kids are stuck eating friggin' two-minute noodles. What the hell is that? It's heartbreaking because it's not poverty of the pocket. It's a poverty of the mind. And that's the thing that motivates me. It motivated me around food sovereignty. (Cherrington 2020)

Her argument was that recent Māori generations, like her parents, were more focused on having a lawn than feeding their children healthy foods because they had been sucked into the colonial, capitalist, model of wealth accumu-lation and ideas of keeping up appearances, regardless of whether they were affordable. More recently, many Māori, Cherrington argues, are more focused on the ability to care for others as being a marker of wealth (2020). Oddom's work on reaching underserved communities through their health care provider is similar to Esquivel's efforts. They share a focus on making healthy food for healthy communities in a culturally appropriate manner. Whereas Oddom's story is more focused on overcoming the neocolonial health care system,

Esquivel's work tries to accomplish similar goals through an economic lens. She asserts:

> Our job is to make our communities healthier, but we've been seeing the same problem for so many years now. We keep telling them, you have to eat this or that. But we know the truth that when they go to the grocery store, that's not realistic if you don't earn a livable wage. In those terms, it's hard to think of a farmer's bottom dollar. (Esquivel 2019)

She understands the necessity of farmers earning a living wage, at the same time as she sees her clients unable to afford local, whole food products because they are not making a livable wage themselves. This vicious cycle perpetuates itself and continues to keep local farmers' profits low, which doesn't entice new farmers into the profession, and continues to encourage local people to buy Spam and Vienna sausage because it is the only thing they can afford, leading to detrimental health outcomes.

Alicia Higa and Moulika Hitchens, from the Waiʻanae Coast Comprehensive Health Center on health promotions and sustainability initiatives, work with Esquivel toward similar goals. Higa argues that being from a particular community makes one attuned to that community's needs. This makes perfect sense, of course, though interestingly, Hitchens, who is not from the Leeward Coast, says she made it her mission to bring in new ideas. In addition, Higa says:

> Basically, I *am* the Health Promotion department. I created this department. I created a food systems program out of a need because I learned that I didn't have to be an expert on what everyone else was an expert. *I became an expert of my community. I know what the community needs. I knew from growing up here.* Just taking my own experiences, I was able to create this program (emphasis added). (Higa 2019)

Like Oddom, Esquivel, Harwood, Cherrington, and Francis, Higa and Hitchens's work is rooted in community. Their insistence on learning *from* community to design health and nutrition programs that will connect with traditionally underserved and marginalized people in their respective areas is aspirational.

> And the reason for me going to school is that actually helped open up my eyes about what injustices were happening out there. You know, growing up here, you just are used to eating that way because that's how it is, and you don't know any

better but by working at the health center, being able to travel to conferences and having exposure to these kinds of things, it really lit that fire in me that made me angry that nobody was doing anything about it out here. (Higa 2019)

Higa explains that even though she was a community expert and knew what the surrounding community needed, her education helped her expand her horizons about other communities facing similar health disparities. She also learned about proven solutions that she might be able to apply in Wai'anae for its residents' benefit: "Kapolei is only like 11 miles away, but you walk in [to the grocery store], you're met with fresh produce and healthy options. You walk into the stores out here; you're met with a liquor department and a deli" (Higa 2019). Higa is well aware of the Leeward Coast's status as a food desert, and she believes it is her role as the health promotion director of the WCCHC to turn this reality into a place that offers fresh, local, seasonal, culturally appropriate produce to its residents. To this end, she has devised myriad ways to address food insecurity in Wai'anae.

So basically, we had to redefine what good food meant and what supporting some people means. If you have a lot of money, you can afford to eat organic and, you know, shop at Whole Foods and Down to Earth. We wrote for a small grant through the local United Way to help us pay for produce. And then for overall family education, we put on these *'ohana* clinics where they're able to get a larger food distribution, but we do cooking demonstrations and teach them how to take this local produce that might be unfamiliar. We take this familiar food that you're getting at the Food Bank and teach you how to stretch your meals and make them healthier. The last one we just did was last week. We fed five hundred-and-eighty-one people dinner. Then after school, [the kids] are able to come and grab these five-pound commodity food bags to take home. Just one night at one location, a distribution only lasted 45 minutes, and we gave out about twelve thousand pounds of food. (Higa 2019)

The sheer capacity of Higa and Hitchens' program is staggering. This shows that there is a clear need for it and that this work is incredibly important and having an impact on the surrounding community. Although neither woman explicitly identified the Leeward Coast as a food desert, there is disparate access to healthy food in that community (Mironesco 2016). That said, Higa and Hitchens choose *not* to focus on that. Rather, they focus on what they *can* do to improve things. I spoke with them prior to the pandemic. However, one of my students did an internship with them as part of her senior capstone experience during the pandemic. She mentioned that according to Higa, the food distribution events had grown in size by about 300% from pre-pandemic days. This indicates that the pandemic exacerbated that community's needs for food, yet Higa and Hitchens' program was able to make sure that some of the food they distributed was from local sources, and that the recipients knew how to cook with the ingredients. Anecdotally, having driven along that coastline around dinner time, the lines at the various fast-food drive thru restaurants are very long. Many community folks work multiple jobs to make ends meet and, at the end of the day, and they are too exhausted to start a dinner from scratch.

This means that recipes and culinary traditions get lost. This does not mean that people should necessarily only adhere to ancient traditions, but that it is important to continue passing down recipes through the generations, as they have been, typically from mothers and aunties to daughters and nieces. Higa and Hitchens' program(s) intend to keep those traditions going. At the same time, budgets are important in decision-making about food. For instance, Joleen Oshiro, the food writer for the *Honolulu Star—Advertiser*, reflected on her audience by saying:

> People are really primarily looking for economy when they cook. We're all trained to think about the canvas bag with the head of cabbage that will feed your whole family for cheap. So many people in my community still cook like that and eat that way because they have to. And that's the kind of approach [my former editor] was catering to when she wasn't writing "white tablecloth" pieces. For her, I think she wondered if it was a little bit pretentious, you know, for me to be talking about all this local food stuff, which was so much more expensive before the farmers' market really took root. (Oshiro 2019)

Oshiro writes about local food for local people, but for decades, local food in Hawaiʻi was hard to find and more expensive than imported foods due to the economies of scale available through food shipping in refrigerated containers. Locally grown food's availability and accessibility has increased in recent years, with the largest growth and interest taking hold during the pandemic. When Hawaiʻi residents realized that it might be difficult, or even dangerous to buy food at the grocery store due to potential exposure to COVID-19, they started growing their own food, and trading fruits and vegetables with neighbors. The number of community supported agriculture (CSAs) and amount of food delivery rose almost exponentially, as it did throughout the nation (Westervelt 2020).

I felt like it was important to pay farmers back in terms by helping them develop new markets maybe or new customers. I'm not sure. I think a lot more people understand what happens when you go to a farmers' market, the ramifications of shopping locally is that you are supporting the farmer directly. I think more people understand that now. I don't know how many, but I think it's more common knowledge than it used to be. It's clear that spending the money at the farmers' market goes directly to the farmer rather than some middleman. (Oshiro 2019)

There must be a balance between keeping people's budgets in mind and pushing potentially more expensive local food to people who cannot afford it. The irony, of course, is that local food *should* be cheaper since it is not shipped 2,500 miles across the ocean.

Nevertheless, Hawai'i's food traditions are in the process of being reclaimed, most famously through the Hawai'i Regional Cuisine movement, started by twelve Hawai'i chefs (all now superstars) in 1991. It was intended to put Hawai'i on the map as a major culinary destination after years of relying on imported ingredients and lackluster recipes (Yamashita 2019). In her exploration of the humble lentil, Ligaya Mischan (2022) argues that "recipes are both living history and cultural archive," and if we lose recipes, we lose stories and cultural identity. In many cases, we may also stand to lose our health. It is important to clarify here that the goal is not to add a third shift of cooking healthy food to women's burdens. Jennifer Szalai and Anne-Marie Slaughter, writing separately argue that the idea of "having it all" is no more than a euphemism for "doing it all." Indeed, the break-the-glass-ceiling, girl-boss, lean-in kind of feminism was a lie (2015). The additional burdens of growing, maintaining, harvesting, cooking, and cleaning food cannot be overstated. It is certainly *not* my intention to assert that the women in this study are doing it all because of some of these aforementioned attitudes, nor that they might be encouraging others to "do it all." In fact, there is a very real danger that in ascribing all this leadership work to women, I run the risk of imposing additional work on them. To be sure, most of these women are working to fix the food system not as an addition to other work, but as part of their regular employment, which is different than if they worked in jobs unrelated to the food system. Through grassroots and community-led practices, they are providing leadership, time, skills, and knowledge in service to repairing a food system that has been used to push disadvantaged people to the margins.

Harmonee Williams, the director of Sustʻāinable Molokaʻi, a food distribution, CSA, and food hub program, explains the importance of figuring out what the community needs.

> We said, "OK, what are we going to tackle first?" Of course, we did a lot of community outreach and really what just kept coming up was the two main areas that we saw as having the most potential for positive impact and direct impact were local food systems and energy independence, both energy efficiency and renewable energy. The food one just really took off and I just found myself really drawn to it. I could really see the importance, especially for this island having a long, amazing history of fighting off development and trying to be self-sufficient as possible. (Williams 2019)

Clearly, community outreach *prior* to implementing nutrition and health programs is a common theme throughout the narratives. Williams shows that Molokaʻi's path to food sovereignty, sustainability, and community nutrition is no different than those we have already encountered on Hawaiʻi Island and Oʻahu in terms of involving community members in decision-making about their own assets and nutrition needs. She explains, "[f]arming and agriculture and eating local food had just helped so many of those goals including open space and taking care of the land and reducing the runoff to the reef and then having economic development that didn't involve tourism" (Williams 2019). Disillusionment with the state's overreliance on tourism is a common theme throughout the Hawaiian archipelago and finding other ways to generate income and preserve important agricultural lands is a central tenet of Williams' narrative.

> My husband was born and raised here, and one of his family's biggest struggles is health with much of it being diet-related. This food system thing just tackles so many of these issues that it just really took off, and it's been my focus since then. So that's kind of kind of how I got to this place of being focused on food systems. (Williams 2019)

Williams claims that her husband's Molokaʻi family's health problems are directly related to a lack of fresh food availability. Their experience is very common, especially among Native Hawaiian families. Williams set out to find systemic ways to encourage the consumption of healthy, locally grown food by making farming profitable through the food hub and CSA. Making the food readily available through delivery, food trucks, and CSA pick-ups is critical to Sustʻāinable

Moloka'i's success. If there are no customers, the farmers don't thrive, and if there are no farmers, the customers don't have access to fresh food.

> We have a mobile market, right? We offer EBT and we offer Double [Up Food] Bucks [also called Da Bux locally]. And the mobile market is a little bit unique. We have an online ordering platform software. Any farmer on island, whether it's produce or the grass-fed beef from our livestock co-op or value-added products from bakers, sauces, etc. anybody can list their products. We ask them to do it by Sunday night and they get to name their quantity and their price and then we add a 30 percent markup to that. We sell out of everything super-fast. Most of our leafy greens and our crops like lettuce, carrots, beets, tomatoes go within the first hour. You can see it on the back-end administration of the website. If you just hit refresh every 30 seconds. That first half hour is like a frenzy. If you put something in your cart and you don't click confirm, it'll disappear from your cart. That's exciting. A lot of people say that's a good problem. You have desire that you supply. But we're nowhere near financial stability so we need to increase our volume. Right now, we're still heavily grant dependent. (Williams 2019)

Sust'āinable Moloka'i's wide variety of programs helps shape the Moloka'i food system into something that works for everyone involved, and Williams' joy in sharing how fast it has grown was palpable. She acknowledges that there is more work to do to make the program sustain itself, and that increasing capacity is a key driver of the next phrase of programming.

> Based on that, our second new program area is really working with farmers to increase their production. The two big needs we've heard from farmers are 1) real specific hands-on training 2) and some start-up capital. We've just gotten two grants. One is an ANA [Administration for Native Americans] and another is a USDA grant for socially disadvantaged farmers and ranchers. We didn't really expect to get both so now we're playing their game because there is a little bit of overlap so we're trying to untangle and make some adjustments. But, yeah, it's a good problem to have. (Williams 2019)

Williams has had success in acquiring large grants from governmental agencies like the USDA, and Moloka'i, with its proportionately large Native Hawaiian population—approximately 63% of about 7,000 residents (Office of Hawaiian Affairs 2024)—is an important space to see what can work to improve nutrition to benefit health and decrease the instances of diet-related diseases.

We had a First Nations grant last year, which was specifically to do a food sovereignty assessment. We interviewed 100 homesteaders. How much local food do you eat? How much local food do you grow? Would you like to grow more? What would you like to grow or produce? What do you need? As a result, we have really specific data which came back saying that that people eat 35 to 40 percent local. But I really don't think that's the case because we asked how many servings of fruits, vegetables per day and it was low. How much of that is local was significantly higher but overall, it's just not that much. However, if you don't hunt or fish or grow food, you just go to the stores. (Williams 2019)

Williams's work on Moloka'i is clearly rooted in her community's needs. She did the front-end work of community outreach to gather data on needs, and received funding based on serving Indigenous peoples and fostering food sovereignty. These grants are an excellent resource, but as she says, they do not last, so it is important to become more self-sufficient, both in funding and in food[3]. Williams's work with the Sust'āinable Moloka'i project is rooted both in health and in growing farmers' capacity to meet the food needs of the island community.

Kristin Albrecht is the director of the Hawai'i Island Food Basket. She has won awards for her service to the island of Hawai'i and its mission to end hunger through innovative anti-hunger programs. Much of her work is a model for others in this field. She has been successful in increasing access to healthy food for food-insecure residents though the "Da Bux" Double Up Food Bucks program. She also implemented a program called Da Box—a CSA specifically for Supplemental Nutrition Assistance Program (SNAP) recipients. Her work reflects an understanding of the need to get healthy food to residents while also valuing farmers' work by paying them a fair price for their products. She asserts:

Da Box is what it's known as now. We are also able to offer produce to our recipients at a lower price to make it affordable because we knew affordable food access was really impacting the way people eat. This was our first project in 2014. It has grown from a handful to 200 families routinely. Right now, it's actually a little over 200 and we buy from about somewhere between 50 and 75 farmers, mostly small. We found our niche is increasing, introducing small or beginning farmers to how to help, how to sell. We're a pretty easy place to sell to people. We hold

---

3. As of this writing, due to the Trump administration's focus on ending diversity, equity and inclusion (DEI) programs that address the needs of Indigenous peoples, minorities, or marginalized communities, many of these programs mentioned throughout this chapter are in jeopardy due to federal funding cuts.

their hands and walk them through how to price, you know. Yes, you do need to wash it before it comes in. There are those little, little details. (Albrecht 2019)

Albrecht's creativity in structuring her programs and administering her grants shows that ingenuity and intentionality are two of the most important characteristics in doing this work, especially for as long as Albrecht has been at it. The work of feeding underserved communities, mostly Black, Indigenous, and People of Color (BIPOC) folks, and helping local farmers with sales within an industrial food system that privileges food from the continent, is nothing short of heroic.

One of the pieces that I feel strongly is so important is the food literacy. You can give people all the fresh produce that they want, but if they don't know what they're eating, if they don't know how to eat it, you're not going to move the dial very much. So we focus on food literacy also. And it started with a newsletter that we put out with recipes and instructions. If it's something that will be out of what you think is "normal," if it's a little more exotic, we make sure that we put instructions about how you would eat it. (Albrecht 2019)

Without nutrition and ingredients education, even giving fresh produce away will not have the desired impact of improved health outcomes for low-income residents. Albrecht's insistence on devising different ways to get information to people about how to cook the foods they are receiving is a critical piece of her organization's success.

We also do a "take a backpack" program in all the schools that are 100 percent free, reduced lunch right before the Christmas holiday, because we know those kids are at really high risk of not having food. And one of the grants I got required that I have three thousand dollars' worth of local food I could put in the backpack. You know, it was next to impossible for me to actually find appropriate food. (Albrecht 2019)

The Hawai'i Island Food Basket focuses on children's nutrition because it understands that the absence of school lunch options for low-income children during school holiday periods has a direct impact on their hunger. The supply side of her programs tends to be volatile, especially with climate change and other disasters, such as Kīlauea's eruption in 2018, which covered 13.7 square miles of farmland in lava, resulting in almost US$28 million in farm losses and destroyed 700 homes (LaJeunesse 2018). A lack of farm capacity to produce enough food to feed residents and visitors is an additional concern.

> We've been talking a lot about how to make this island more food secure. And it's not going as fast as we want. One of the big deals is replacing rice with some other form of starch. We have a farmer who started growing potatoes. Everybody said you couldn't grow potatoes in the field. But she is growing the most fabulous little potatoes, which is super exciting. And because we have all the climates here except for one, we should be able to do that. We were just brainstorming this morning how cool it would be if we could get potato bags. They either make them in burlap or so that you can grow them in the bags. If we could write a grant to get, say, a thousand potato bags and give them out to families that we know would really like another source of carbs, maybe replacing the rice and see if we could get potato growing happening, with potato or cassava. (Albrecht 2019)

Again, Albrecht's work has received awards and been used as a model for others doing similar work on other islands and communities on Hawai'i Island. Her leadership demonstrates that women's networks and connections support and lift each other's work up, so that all their projects, and thereby their respective communities may thrive.

Understanding the connection between people, food, and land is central to women's leadership in food system change. Feeding people is a part of what women have traditionally done for millennia. As much as it has been a limiting factor for much of that time, relegating women to fires, stoves, and kitchens, it is also a transformative space for creativity, community, and resistance. Kristin Albrecht uses her creativity in crafting programs that will place local food in Hawai'i Island's most vulnerable communities. She explains that this is "part of the resilience. You have to know what it is you're eating. You have to know how it's grown, and that empowerment comes from both of those things" (Albrecht 2019). Using food as a mechanism of empowerment for vulnerable communities is central to fostering strength. She thus explains how the programs she runs work:

> It is basically aimed at getting out into the rural communities that make up so much of our island and providing healthy food access for those families that live in those areas at a very affordable price. We purchase from our same group of wonderful small farmers and go out and set up basically a mobile basket of local farmers' markets all over the island to make sure that people can access

those fruits and vegetables. And we target the [food deserts]. We actually have 12 USDA designated food deserts, also known as low-income, low-access areas on this island. Those are the target areas for the market.

It's thirty-two dollars for a month of produce. And it's a really nice box. We usually have seven to eight items in it, and it's balanced between staples and then one what could be termed "exotic item" or something really fun to learn about. And we're doing that with Hawaiʻi Island grown produce. All of our programs to date have done Hawaiʻi Island grown produce only. And at all seven of the KTA superstores, 24/7, offer this up and you can buy whatever it is that's marked with the Double Bucks, and it will be half price. It's a one for one. This is a 50 percent discount if you have a SNAP card, an EBT card. (Albrecht 2019)

The specifics of Albrecht's Food Basket program are instructive here, as is the precision with which she understands the communities her work serves. Often, we think of food-insecure places as urban areas with few or no grocery stores for example. As Albrecht explains, vast rural areas like those on Hawaiʻi Island also have limited access to healthy local food, and serving them requires some creative logistical maneuvers.

On Hawaiʻi Island everybody worked so well together. There's just a lack of ego. People really believe in food security and want to make this happen and it became a reality.

Yeah, it's interesting because I think that the women I know who were involved in this work, they love to garden, they love to cook, they love to feed people. I would say that is a common theme if I think about the women involved. But good men, too. I would say that there is real love and passion for food, for food and people, feeding people, and quality food and fairness. I think that the other piece is an urgency for a lot of us who are moms or grandmothers. It's just this next generation. *The current food that's accessible to people is essentially poisoned so changing that requires, I think, insurgency and a dedication that women are really good at doing* (emphasis added). (Albrecht 2019)

Working with community enables Albrecht's organization to accomplish its mission successfully. She credits the women she works with for getting the job done. Like other interviewees for this book, she sees their roles as mothers or grandmothers as a shared experience that drives them to ensure families are fed around the island, regardless of income or location.

What's exciting here in this state, and I will say for Hawai'i Island is that there is no reason we can't make this a super food secure place. There is no reason we cannot actually produce everything that we need here in order to thrive. We've got storage, we've got freezers, we've got refrigeration. We've got trucks that are moving things around. (Albrecht 2019)

Albrecht is passionate about her work, and she recognizes the passion in the other women and players she works with to create and run these programs. Most interestingly, she recognizes the need for resistance to the status quo fostering creativity in changing the food system.

Managing long-term health conditions makes the most sense from a preventative perspective. Dr. Matire Harwood does exactly that in South Auckland. She explains that "the evidence has shown that once Māori and Pacific peoples leave the hospital to go home, they deteriorate compared to non-Māori Pacific people. So we got a whole group of long-term condition and diabetes experts together. We wanted to look at addressing diabetes with a focus on equity" (Harwood 2020). Understanding barriers to healthcare access and social determinants of health, Dr. Harwood and her team at the Papakura Marae Health Clinic aim to reduce the numbers of Pacific peoples with chronic diseases through nutrition education and encouragement of physical activity to improve family well-being. She shared the story of a woman who was too ashamed to go walk outside because of her weight (Harwood 2020) but through talking story with others in similar situations, was able to overcome her shame and walk outside to exercise and improve her health. By bringing people together and sharing stories through a program called Oranga ki Tua, they foster a sense of community of healthy practices. This work is not without its difficulties, however. When residents of South Auckland can get

fried chicken and chips for $5NZ, whereas to get a loaf of bread, and some tomatoes and a salad will be $20NZ. It's miles to walk to this main supermarket with cheaper food too. Poverty drives a lot of the issues that we see. Oh sorry, did I say [out loud]? (Harwood 2020)

Harwood focuses on improving health outcomes in marginalized communities living below the poverty line in food-insecure urban areas. Similarly, Clifford works to "connect agriculture and food experience. To help eaters find their farmers and fishers, and vice versa. To grow food communities" (Clifford 2020). While Clifford's focus is likely to be people with the privilege to make decisions about their health and diet that are *not* based on cost but rather on experience, the notion of growing food communities is an excellent stepping stone for food system reform to serve *all* eaters.

Conclusion

The connection between nutritious food and environmental sustainability is integral to a healthy food system. It must also include access to culturally appropriate foods, thereby reclaiming our food systems from corporate-owned industrial giants. Re-regionalizing our food systems will enable us to grow healthier and more resilient food systems and distribute healthy food to our most marginalized communities. But there must be a systemic policy focus to enable these changes to foster food sovereignty. We cannot solely rely on business or nonprofit organizations to make these things happen. There is hope in the examples discussed here of school food programs, as well as food pantry and health clinic distributions of local food with cooking instructions for low-income families. However, their lasting impact would be well-served by policy and legislative support. At this point, these businesses and nonprofit organizations are only as strong as the economy and the potentially tenuous grant-funding that support them. Structural support through a politico-legal framework would serve to improve the food systems in Hawai'i and Aotearoa New Zealand to provide locally grown, culturally appropriate foods to greater numbers of people throughout their respective islands.

CHAPTER 5

Weighing the Values of Plant-Based Diets and Local Meat, Fish, and Dairy Production and Consumption

Indigenous people believe we were born of all these creatures. The rocks are our grand-fathers. The plants are our grandmothers. And all the animals are the parents of humanity.
—T'uy't'tanat-Cease Wyss (2019)

Producing and Consuming Meat, Fish, and Dairy

Much of the discussion throughout the book has centered on local fruit and vegetable production and consumption. I interviewed three women working in the meat, fishing, and dairy industries who have carved out niches for themselves in this sector by creating innovative models for harvesting, processing, and distributing their products: Jessica Rohr, who owns and operates Forage Hawai'i, which sells locally-sourced meats and meat-derived value added products to local eaters; Ashley Watts, executive director of Local 'Ia, which she describes as a community-supported fishery (CSF), a fishing cooperative in Hawai'i; and Cathy Tait-Jameson, the co-owner of BioFarm, an organic dairy farm in Palmerston North, on the North Island of Aotearoa New Zealand. I did not have an opportunity to interview Michelle Galimba, the co-owner and vice president of Kuahiwi Ranch on Hawai'i Island but many would agree that Galimba is one of the leading figures in this domain. After earning her PhD in comparative literature at the University of California, Berkeley (UC Berkeley), she came back to her home in Ka'ū to help her family run a cattle ranch. According to the ranch website, the family currently lease 10,000 acres of pastureland on the southern tip of Hawai'i Island, where they raise approximately 3,000 head of cattle. The margins for this operation are razor thin, so efficiency is the key to success. In multiple interviews available online, Galimba explained that in the 1990s, it became almost impossible to grow and finish cattle in Hawai'i. Due to the closure of processing facilities, cattle had to be shipped to the continent for fattening and slaughtering, and then shipped back to Hawai'i, processed, and boxed up for sale. Ethanol subsidies and the increased cost of fuel for shipping raised the cost of corn for forage, making this model unsustainable; yet, Hawai'i's dependence on imported meat continues (https://kuahiwi.com/). Kuahiwi Ranch markets their products to high-end restaurants on O'ahu, as well as locally owned grocery stores, yet they still cannot meet the demand for local beef.

Jessica Rohr aims to build on that model and increase the diversity of local meat available in Hawai'i. Rohr studied nutrition and business at the University of Hawai'i at Mānoa, yet did not believe that the USDA recommendations for a nutritious diet were sound. At that time, the push was "low fat everything is good for you" (Rohr 2019). She explains the process as follows:

> Through my [UH nutrition] education, I found that the government is basically giving us recommendations based on what the industry is paying them to lobby. I was totally turned off by that, but I did learn about the importance of the nutrition that we get from animal products. I was vegetarian because I've always been against factory farming, so it's been a drive not only to eat locally for food security but to know where my food comes from and to know what's put on it and know how it's raised. That's the part that I appreciate about it. That's why I try and go and see the slaughterhouses and visit all these places. (Rohr 2019)

Rohr's focus on the ethics of eating local meat is important in the larger context of a food system that privileges factory-grown and imported meat. She takes the time to know her ranchers and visits the slaughterhouses so that she can share the information with her consumers, educate them on the importance of eating local meat, meet their nutritional needs, and eradicate invasive species like axis deer and feral pigs.

> All the nutrients that you need, especially from animal foods, you can't get from plant foods. It's sad and painful because I just feel like there is a lack of knowledge. With ancestral wisdom, we had so much knowledge in terms of how our food supported pregnancy and women's health and we've just forgotten that. I see so much information out there that's just making people assume that they can just drink soy milk and eat plant-based and then they're going to be healthy. And then you see 10, 15 years later, these people have major health problems. (Rohr 2019)

Rohr credits Indigenous foodways for their wisdom in including meat products in their diets. She highlights the importance of meat in women's diets to supplement iron intake. Her experience as a former vegetarian and new mother sharpened the urgency of her mission.

> The customers get mad at you for not having what they want. It's like, man, we're trying our best to make this available. Sometimes it's hard because you don't feel as appreciated. People don't know how much work [it is] to get all these different things to the customer. I think I have probably the best variety of anyone selling local meat.
>
> At least they can support local farms. It's unclear why we don't have our EBT money pushing our local meat staying in Hawai'i. Instead of buying all this mainland product, we can look at comparisons whether this meat is better for you. We know it's better for the land and it's better for the environment. (Rohr 2019)

Sustainability issues associated with growing and processing meat, as well as the nutritional aspects of a diverse diet, drive Rohr's mission to get more local meat onto the plates of Hawai'i residents. Being a woman in this space has proven to be a difficult but not insurmountable obstacle. She explains that she is inspired by powerful women doing work at high levels. She even speculates that some of the negative stereotypes about women having an iron deficiency could be addressed by eating more red meat:

> It's one of the reasons nutrition is really important to me and meat is really important to me, because although red meat and steaks are kind of associated with a man's food, women need those nutrients more than men. Our requirement for iron is higher. It relates to my nutrition background. A lot of the symptoms of iron deficiency are related some of the stereotypes about women like absent-minded, forgetful, not strong, weak types. (Rohr 2019)

Rohr's discussion of the gendered aspects of meat consumption is instructive here. She argues that eating meat is associated with men, but that women should be consuming more of it to meet their nutritional needs. Her nutrition background explains her insistence on this issue, and she finds herself in an interesting position as a woman in a male-dominated industry, trying to get more women to eat more meat.

Meat, of course, is not the only protein available in Hawai'i; we are surrounded by the Pacific Ocean. Fishing has its roots in Indigenous traditions and was an important source of protein for Kanaka Maoli populations on all the islands since the ahupuaʻa land management system included access to near-shore and deep-sea fishing with ocean-going canoes. Different kinds of fishing traditions represented the different strengths of the population. Hawaiians had an ingenious system of *loko ʻia* (traditional Hawaiian fishponds), in which near-shore fish came to breed and grow in brackish water adjacent to the shoreline and grew too large to exit out of the *makahā* (gates) built into the rock walls at regular intervals. This made for easy fishing and required a scientific understanding of the ecosystem and the lifecycles of different fish species (Innes-Gold, et al 2024). As Hiʻilei Kawelo, the Executive Director of Paepae O Heʻeia Fishpond explains (Kawelo 2016), society has lost the taste for these near-shore herbivorous fish because they taste "fishy." Instead, everyone is interested in large predatory, deep-sea fish like ahi (tuna), mahi mahi (dolphinfish), or ono (wahoo). Kawelo explains that to be sustainable and promote local fish consumption, we must retrain our palates to value fish grown in loko ʻia to avoid depleting deep-sea fish stocks due to our insatiable demand for large fish species.

To address this issue, Ashley Watts who took over Local ʻIa, converted its business model to mimic a CSA scheme. She calls it a CSF—a community supported fishery. This model prevents overfishing because

> Even if they keep catching fish, sometimes they don't even have enough ice. Then the value of the fish is so bad that they can't sell it for a good price even if they have enough access. If people just whack the whole population of a certain school that comes in, the market's not going to buy all of them. (Watts 2019)

Watts focuses on the sustainability aspect of fisheries management not only due to her biology background, but also because it just makes better business sense not to flood the market with too many fish since it will drive down the price for each fisher. Additionally, Hawaiian waters are already overfished as fish populations have declined by 75% (Bergman 2020).

> I came into this organization having been a fisher my whole life and having friends and family who produce their food. Prior to me joining, they were just a subscription service. They were just buying fish for that, which made it really hard for fishermen to be able to sell them fish because they only wanted this very little amount every weekend. If you're a fisherman, you have a certain amount and if somebody is only going to buy a little bit, that makes more work because he's going to go somewhere else to try to sell his fish.

The first thing I needed to do is to create more outlets for the fish so I can buy more fish. Then I also saw the need to be able to market myself and to be able to have an outlet to increase sales and have a way to get rid of a lot more fish. It's all just seeing how things work and figuring out ways to maintain the income, to cover the expenses and to get more fishermen. I have probably 50 guys who sell me fish. (Watts 2019)

Increasing Local 'Ia's capacity to distribute more fish to more people and restaurants became an important tool to support her fishers and their livelihoods at the same time as she encourages fishers to be sustainable by not overfishing and providing avenues for value-added fish product production and sales.

To create a value-added product, we've developed a product called Fish Crack. It's dried ahi. And it's super *ono* [good, tasty]. It's not only like selling their fish, but helping them sustain themselves through other means, too. If we could get them set up as a value-added fisherman, that would be a really true market success on our part because we would be able to provide something for the fisherman to sustain himself, instead of having to sell his fish on the street. So in this way, he'd be able to make money when the fish were biting, and this product is one where you can take the fish and freeze it and make the product after. So even when there's a surplus, we can also take advantage of that. (Watts 2019)

Watts works with fisher folks to create avenues for selling their fish at the same time as she guarantees them a certain price because the fish has already been sold through the CSF model. This helps the fishers avoid overfishing because once they have reached the price Local 'Ia is paying for the day, they can just come back to the harbor instead of continuing to fish and deplete the fishery. With high fuel prices in 2022, this option became even more attractive. Sustainability is a key goal for the CSF model and has wide ranging implications for Hawai'i fisheries, especially if more people are willing to buy from Local 'Ia and other similar entities. Local 'Ia partnered with Farm Link Hawai'i, which increases access to a large consumer base, as well as providing an option for local fish for SNAP and EBT users both at farmers' markets and through the Farm Link Hawai'i website. These kinds of innovative models and partnerships enable these businesses to thrive while they are putting a local protein option in local residents' kitchens. It also enables fisher folks to anticipate demand so that they can calibrate supply and avoid overfishing. This moves us toward decentralizing the Hawai'i food system and encouraging sustainable micro-regional food systems that work within smaller geographic regions, similarly to the ahupua'a system of old.

Māori fishing traditions in Aotearoa New Zealand echo those found in the Hawaiian archipelago, though admittedly with some significant differences. Unfortunately, I was not able to interview anyone with specific fishery experience in order to provide qualitative evidence for any similarities or differences. However, fishing was, and remains, a significant part of the food system in Aotearoa New Zealand. Per the Fisheries New Zealand government website "fishing rights for Māori are guaranteed by New Zealand law. Customary fisheries are recognized fishing rights of tangata whenua (people of the land with authority in a particular place) and the rights are guaranteed through legislation" (Ministry for Primary Industries 2025). Māori fishing practices took advantage of abundant near-shore fishing stocks, which provided them with a rich source of protein. Furthermore, eels were an important source of Māori cultural foodways (Paulin 2007) and remain important today as symbols of reclaiming Māori identity and pride through foodways. While there is some debate about whether Aotearoa New Zealand's fisheries management is as robust in supporting sustainability as it should be (Melnychuk et al. 2017; Slooten et al. 2017), given the fact that the islands are surrounded by ocean, using fish as a source of protein is a common practice throughout Oceania. Increasing accessibility to fish for balanced and healthy diets is an important practice and must be weighed against sustainable fisheries management. Māori iwi and hapū have access to specific fishing grounds surrounding their traditional lands through the formal governance structures of the 1992 Māori Fisheries Settlement (Te Ohu Kaimoana 2017). They rely on traditional Indigenous practices to manage their own fisheries, some for profit, and some for subsistence of the whānau in the surrounding areas. The fisheries settlement provides a mechanism for Māori to develop their own governance over fishing activities, which contribute to the health of their respective communities. Given the settlement's focus on restoring fisheries to iwi organizations, Māori voices are valued in fisheries management in Aotearoa New Zealand, forging a path toward food sovereignty. This is vastly different compared to the Hawai'i situation, whereby the food system relies on the private development of cooperatives like Watts's Local 'Ia, or nonprofit loko 'ia restoration projects to provide fish for community consumption and to educate fishers and consumers on sustainable fisheries. While these are valuable inroads toward food sovereignty and the restoration of Indigenous foodways in Hawai'i, they are not supported by legal precedents as they are in Aotearoa New Zealand.

Small-scale, sustainable dairy farms respond to environmentally damaging industrialized dairy operations. On O'ahu, there are two small dairies run by women, none of whom I was able to interview unfortunately. Sweetland Farms on the north shore is owned by Emma Bello who grew up just up the road in Wāhiawa and spent a summer working at Maui's famous Surfing Goat Dairy. It consists of 86 acres of old pineapple land. Bello and her family manage a herd of about 100 goats for dairy production and other goat milk products like soaps, lotions, a variety of cheeses, and caramels. The farm also conducts tours and field trips to expose children to farm animals. Naked Cow Dairy, in Wai'anae, recently opened another dairy farm on Hawai'i Island. It was founded by the van der Stroom sisters. *Food and Wine* profiled the dairy in a 2018 article praising its women-run, non-hierarchical business practices (Sherman). Naked Cow's commitment to rebuilding small local dairy capacity in the face of cheap imported milk is exemplary. Gupta argues that "the trajectory of milk production in Hawai'i has precluded the survival of regionalized milksheds" (2018), meaning that it is more cost-effective to import milk from the US continent. However, the owners of Naked Cow Dairy focus on processing their own value-added products in order to cater to local food tastes and interests and avoid the fluid milk prices set artificially low by the Hawai'i Milk Act of 1967.

Cathy Tait-Jameson's experience in Aotearoa New Zealand stemmed from taking over her husband's family dairy farm, where the animals were stressed and getting sick due to conventional agricultural practices. Her family reframed their agricultural practices to reflect biodynamic practices following the teachings of Rudolph Steiner and focused on "creating food that was good for people, but also good for the environment and the animals" (Tait-Jameson 2020). The conventional way to farm dairy cows is to milk year-round, but they saw that as unsustainable. Additionally, to buy out her husband's family, they needed to add value to the milk, so they worked with a local dairy company that made yogurt. Because their milk was organic, the dairy company agreed, and they started making yogurt out of BioFarm's milk. They started a market garden as well that provided produce to a large health food store in Wellington, but their yogurt took off and their dairy operation grew so much that they now have to buy milk from other producers to keep up with the demand. The farm has thrived and become a model of a sustainable dairy farm, which is a feat in Aotearoa New Zealand, considering its many polluted waterways and the environmental impacts of its large conventional meat and dairy operations. Tait-Jameson told me that she saw dairy farming as a gendered occupation. Although it is traditionally associated with men, she thought women might be more capable at it because caring for dairy cows is like caring for family.

> I feel like the animal farming is definitely more male-dominated than vegetable farming. I don't know why that is, because as I see it, it's like having a family. There are a lot of women in agriculture in New Zealand, but they're just not at the forefront. I'd say a lot of farms would be run by women. But I think we're here. We're really resilient. You just get knocked down, but you keep getting right back up. I think if we believe in something strongly enough, we just keep coming back. (Tait-Jameson 2020)

Her understanding of the animals as part of a family erases the hierarchical distinction between her dairy cows and humans. They are all part of the same family. This ethos is rooted in her Māori heritage, which, similarly to the Native Hawaiian view, sees humans are deeply embedded in nature and everything around us. Tait-Jameson took a lighthearted approach, joking that raising dairy cows was like having children; impossible to go on vacation without having someone to care for the cows so that they would remain happy and produce high-quality milk. She showed me around the operation and shared how the pasture rotation kept the cows grazing on the highest nutrient grass for their benefit as well as for the higher quality of milk they produce, which in turn leads to her highly prized value-added yogurt. This holistic understanding of the farm's ecosystem is rooted in a combination of her Māori upbringing, her education about Steiner's biodynamic principles as applied to dairy farming, and her appreciation for the Native American ideals of gift giving to her surroundings (Tait-Jameson 2020).

Comparing this kind of sustainable farming with the practices at Fonterra, one of Aotearoa New Zealand's largest corporations in one of the largest industries in the country, is stark. Most of Fonterra's dairy is exported to China in the form of whole milk powder (Hancock 2021b), for revenue of US$14.04 billion in 2021 (Companies Market Cap 2025). This statistic reveals the chasm between farming for corporate profits and feeding community. Although Fonterra's share of the dairy market decreased from 96% in 2001 to 82% in 2019, their impact on Aotearoa New Zealand's GDP is still 3% and accounts for over 20% of exports (New Zealand Productivity Commission 2020). Each kind of dairy farming has very different environmental impacts: large-scale dairy farming pollutes waterways and contributes to soil erosion and ocean degradation (Naranjo et al. 2020) while small-scale and regional dairy farming regenerates soil health (Chrisman

2025; Voth and Gilker 2017). As Hancock describes "ninety-five percent of New Zealand's dairy is exported, but the country still has to deal with 100% of cows' urine and feces, as well as the excess chemicals from fertiliser [sic] for their feed leaching into waterways" (2021a). Like those of Rohr and Watts presented earlier, Tait-Jameson's philosophies all work together to create sustainable farming practices that produce healthy food available to people in her community without the deleterious environmental impacts that large agribusinesses and factory farming are prone to inflicting on their surroundings.

The Intersectional Politics of Producing and Consuming Meat, Fish, and Dairy

Intersectional feminism has been used in the feminist food studies literature to both condemn and support plant-based diets based on various applications and interpretations. FPE suggests that there is nothing inherently wrong with producing and consuming meat, fish, and/or dairy products (Hovorka 2023), but that the current industrialized factory farming model of protein production is fundamentally problematic. Indeed, as Carol Adams argued in *The Sexual Politics of Meat* (1990), it reproduces patriarchy through the objectification of animals so that they are rendered "being-less" and once objectified can be consumed. Proponents of various plant-based diets ranging from vegetarianism to veganism argue that the production and consumption of animal products reproduces patriarchal relations. As Adams notes (1990), meat-eating can be construed as a masculine endeavor that reproduces power and privilege. Environmentally, those most affected by the externalities of factory farming tend to be marginalized peoples and communities—most often consisting of people of color and/or Indigenous peoples. In this view, meat production and consumption contribute to the deleterious effects of industrialized agriculture, leading to climate change through methane emissions and deforestation, waterway pollution, and other environmental hazards. According to vegan ecofeminist Greta Gaard, intersectionality goes beyond the various "isms" of oppression like sexism, heterosexism, racism, classism, etc., to include speciesism as well. She argues that industrialized animal agriculture reinforces binary gender roles that disproportionately exploits animals designated as females for their bodily secretions such as milk and eggs (Gaard 1993; Gaard 2013). This view, however, is not universal.

Even though industrialized animal agriculture accounted for some 14.5% of greenhouse gas emissions globally in 2013 (UN Food and Agriculture

Organization), some feminist food studies scholars see the industrialized aspect of animal agriculture as problematic, rather than animal agriculture in and of itself. Kathy Rudy (2011) argues that society should instead rely on small-scale, sustainable farming practices that enable better treatment of other species and raise the standards of care for growing animals for food. Temple Grandin (2021) provides another perspective on farming animals that includes considerations of their needs as they are killed for human consumption. However, all of these approaches have one thing in common: they tend to avoid examining their whiteness or their privilege. As Davis et al. (2022) explain, transforming food systems to support plant-based diets that eliminate all meat and dairy products risks further disadvantaging the rural poor globally because they might rely on animal husbandry and/or hunting to ensure both their livelihoods or perhaps their family's subsistence. Julie Guthman (2007, 2011) has taken the alternative food movement to task for privileging a certain upper-middle-class, white, urban perspective to the detriment of marginalized communities by reproducing what Gillespie calls "racialized, colonial social relations when they enter communities of color and implement food practices that ignore cultural and racial histories" (2018, 156). They also ignore the lived experiences of poor, Black/Brown folks who may not have the financial capacity to participate in plant-based diets or in the alternative food movement, or simply do not have the means to purchase more expensive, non-government subsidized foods like fresh local vegetables. Asking folks in marginalized communities to eat less meat to reduce climate impacts while more privileged communities have easier access to healthy, pasture-raised meats reproduces inequality. These problematic perspectives hinder inclusive food system transformation in many ways.

Veganism as a practice that tends to be associated with white people can erase cultural differences, especially when it comes to Indigenous foods. Isaias Hernandez (2022), a self-described vegan environmental educator spreading his message through social media (@queerbrownvegan on Instagram) describes "White Veganism as a form of veganism that focuses solely on animal liberation while actively ignoring the effects of colonization and how it is connected to the oppression of humans and animals." He argues that a more inclusive veganism is inherently anti-colonial, anti-imperialist, and anti-capitalist, and that solutions combining the anti-racist calls of BIPOC vegans must be local and rooted in community, accountability, and justice. Solutions should be rooted in the lived experiences of the people in the affected communities and should focus on the assets they bring to the food system. It is too simplistic to label certain communities as marginalized, without acknowledging that there are "intersectional differentiations even within these groups that are shaped by broader structural and institutional inequalities" (Tavenner et al. 2022, 386) that predicate access to plant-based diet options. In an interview with *Passerby Magazine*, Claudia Serrato, an Indigenous plant-based chef and culinary anthropologist, finds that avoiding the language of veganism altogether is most effective in discussing plant-based diets because of its association with what she calls "ideologies of white racial purity" (2021). Avoiding prescriptive diets, strict culinary rules, and alternative food labels, and instead focusing on food and ecosystems as relatives sharing and giving ancestral wisdom and nourishment, constitutes the way forward for many Indigenous food system scholars and activists.

This may look different in Oceania than in the continental United States, and it may encompass different environmental justice practices in urban and rural areas. For example, Māori and Kanaka Maoli both have long-standing fishing traditions, and both communities eat meat and a variety of seafoods regularly. Māori traditionally hunted a wide range of birds and ate (and still eat) mussels and eels. The Kanaka Maoli diet included pigs as well. These traditional foods remain staples of communities in both places that are reclaiming their traditional foodways. This process of decolonizing diets reconnects Indigenous communities to sustainable agricultural practices rooted in Indigenous knowledge. As Michelle Daigle (2017) explains, this work connects contemporary Indigenous communities with ancestral foodways and relationships to land to promote healing from colonial violence. There is no single view of meat- or fish-eating practices from Indigenous perspectives, of course, and there are Indigenous vegans, such as Margaret Robinson, who writes (2013) that an ethic of care for the land includes caring for animals by *not* killing and eating them, nor by using the milk for dairy products that would be meant for their babies. Be it from an Indigenous, feminist, or vegan perspective, most can agree that there should be less industrialized agriculture, and more care for animal well-being, environmental sustainability, and reducing the climate impacts of animal agriculture.

One of the highlights of traditional ecological knowledge based on Indigenous foodways is the agricultural understanding of how nature and humans work together within ecosystems. Nature necessarily includes animals. These agricultural practices are not limited to Indigenous food systems. Famous for his starring roles in Michael Pollan's *Omnivore's Dilemma*, the 2009 award-winning documentary film *Food, Inc.* among many other popular culture venues, Joel Salatin of

Polyface Farms in Virginia, argues that sustainable farming must mimic natural patterns, which themselves include animals. Plant-based diets ignore the many roles animals play in nature: providing ecosystem services, converting grass to protein for human consumption, and participating in diversified ecosystems. The problematic presence of invasive species (both plant and animal) in isolated ecosystems like those of Hawai'i and Aotearoa New Zealand adds an extra layer to the issues of diversified and regenerative agricultural systems. Hawai'i is colloquially known as the "endangered species capital of the world" due to invasive species destruction of Native habitats (Kunze 2023), and Aotearoa New Zealand has instituted some of the strictest customs inspections in the world to avoid following the same path.

Laurie Carlson, one of the grand dames of Hawai'i's sustainable food scene, was instrumental in starting the Slow Food Hawai'i chapter and was a founding member of the Kokua Market Cooperative. She views alternative food movements as a pendulum swing from industrialized processed foods to what she calls a "natural food ecosystem" (Carlson 2019). When she started with Kokua Market, a natural foods cooperative, she explains that "the whole idea was to get away from processed foods and industrialized foods as much as anything and to control our own food, supply our diets, and make good choices" (Carlson 2019). But she decries the current state of natural foods stores in general, with their emphasis on industrialized and processed vegan options. Agribusiness is using this foodway moment to market these products to a younger generation of environmentally conscious consumers, but these artificial meat-substitute imitation foods essentially increase corporate control over food and perpetuate the centralized food system. These foods do not address the inherent problems with industrial agriculture. Indeed, she condemns the food industry for capitalizing on people's attitudes toward "natural foods":

> What I see has happened is people who are vegans go and create processed foods or industrialized foods. How does it come back with a vengeance? If you want gluten free, we'll manufacture 5,000 products like mac and cheese so that you can eat organic, industrialized food. The industry just has its claws right back in to where we started because they're looking at marketability and profit possibilities. And they put all the "right" names on their products. It's really just mindboggling to me that these young people then fall for it. It's like just putting out cans of fake meat, Vienna sausage made from plants. Why wouldn't you just have some zucchini? Why do we have to go there? We should just teach kids how to cook real food. (Carlson 2019)

It is unclear whether people are simply "falling for it" or whether the marketing capabilities of the industrial agro-food system are so strong that they are impossible to avoid. Nevertheless, Carlson's experience shows that there was once a focus on cooking whole foods from scratch. She asserts that it was the women who "played that role in the kitchen from their mothers' time and it wasn't a far reach to say, 'hey this is something that I'm passionate about and interested in and since I do the cooking, I want to change the way I cook and get the right ingredients' " (Carlson 2019). The "right ingredients" in today's Hawai'i foodscape can be found either at various farmers' markets or through CSA schemes based on different models and may well contain locally sourced or produced meat or fish-based proteins.

Practical applications of cooperative and Indigenous knowledge-led approaches to protein production and consumption both in Aotearoa New Zealand and in Hawai'i can be employed in a solutions-based framework to address problems within the food system. For example, Rohr and Forage Hawai'i support local farmers and ranchers in reducing Hawai'i's reliance on imported foods by responding to what Rohr calls the "visibly obvious problem" of invasive axis deer on the island of Maui: "they're everywhere on the island." Axis deer were brought to Hawai'i in the 1860s as a gift from Hong Kong to King Kamehameha V. The original group of animals consisted of only eight deer. Yet because there are no natural predators for axis deer in Hawai'i, there are now approximately 50,000 axis deer on Maui; about 70,000 on Moloka'i, where there are only about 7,000 residents; and 25,000 on Lāna'i, which has a population of just 3,100 people (Heaton 2022). They cause millions of dollars of damage every year. Their foraging habits cause erosion, which impacts the watershed. They eat Native plants, sometimes to the brink of extinction, causing formerly lush landscapes to become desert-like, which in turn impacts Native insects and birds (Nosowitz 2021). Their herds are also so large that they knock down cattle fencing so that they can graze unrestricted, to the detriment of existing cattle on ranches on all of these islands. Clearly, finding ways to curtail these populations is an important priority. Finding markets for venison to reduce the axis deer population is part of Forage Hawai'i's mission.

Rohr works with Maui Nui Venison, a Maui-based company whose mission statement is to "help balance axis deer populations for the food of our environment, communities and food systems" (Maui Nui Venison 2025). She intends to help their venison products reach more consumers. Her original goal, she says, was

> just to make local meat more available and then just educate people about healthy ways to eat meat. [At Maui Nui Venison] they really respect the resource, even

though it's invasive and not just exploit it. The goal is not just to make money...I was just focused on selling the venison but there's really low margins
in the meat and meat sales. [Most importantly] people have to start eating this
way more because it is a solution to the factory farm meat issue. (Rohr 2019)

Rohr's work addresses several problems with the unsustainable food system in
Hawai'i at once: she sells invasive venison and provides access to local meat
for consumers; she helps another business distribute their products on neighbor
islands, increasing their reach; she is not focused simply on profit, but also on
the environmental and nutritional benefits of eating wild game.

Rohr explains that, due to consumer habits of getting what we want when we
want it, she has encountered customers getting upset because she has run out
of certain products. She says she doesn't feel appreciated sometimes, because

> people don't know how much work goes in to get all these different items to the
> markets...[But] I think the more people connect with their food source, the more
> they respect it, the more there is a benefit to have a better understanding about
> the circle of life. For us to live, something has to have died no matter what. If
> you were to go to a factory farm that was doing plants, you would see the loss
> of ecosystems, the loss of native species, the loss of animals that die from their
> tractors and the pesticides. And you might be more understanding about an open
> pasture with animals that are converting grass that we can't utilize into high
> quality protein. (Rohr 2019)

Even though her customers are mostly millennial women, she says, they will
look right past her at the farmers' market and ask if "he [the owner]" is there,
because they associate ranching, fishing, dairying, and butchering with men.
In these environments, however, women show up to support each other's work
and amplify each other's voices. Rohr admires women working in similarly
male-dominated fields and hopes to inspire other women business owners in
the food sector. She says that

> the camaraderie is important because when women get together and are doing
> something like this, it's so beneficial. I think we all probably second guess
> ourselves. You look at the differences in how men see themselves and their con-
> fidence compared to women. We just naturally tend to be less confident so when
> we get together as supporters for each other, we thrive. I've kind of just powered
> through it on my own. You have to be able to sell. You have to be able to take

money from people and know your value. When you lack the self-confidence to
do that, it's really hard. It was so stressful for me for the longest time but now I
have fun with it. (Rohr 2019)

Many of the women in this study, especially the younger ones, expressed that
they suffered from "imposter syndrome," a phenomenon whereby successful
people do not feel like they deserve to be where they are or that they somehow
haven't earned their positions. Rohr articulates this sense when she says that she
often second guesses herself and explains that talking story with other women
helps everyone lift their experiences up. Here, women's intentionality supports
other women and fosters their respective agency to successfully complete the
necessary work of repairing the food system.

Imposter syndrome among women working in AFNs is also prevalent because
suppliers/producers sometimes express doubt. It is not just farmers' market
consumers who mistakenly assume that the owner of Forage Hawai'i is a man.
For example, Watts explained that the fishers she worked with initially didn't
have faith in her or her business model simply because it was different than what
they were used to. She insisted on paying them a fair price for high-quality fish
in order to maintain fish stocks in the region, rather than encouraging them to
fish as much as possible so that they could sell higher quantities of fish, even
lower-quality fish, for a lower price.

> Through Local 'Ia, we source fish and seafood directly and distribute it to con-
> sumers and chefs around the island directly to shorten the supply chain to give
> the fishermen more money and the consumer product. This also creates a value
> on the resource and treats it as a resource and not a commodity. The price is based
> on the value of the resource. We pay the fishermen a fair wage all year round that
> way they can go out and catch fish and know what they're getting paid so they
> can stop catching fish after a certain number of hours. We've actually seen an
> improvement over the years that we've been doing it, and we have more fishermen
> calling and asking how many fish we need and actually stopping fishing once
> they've reached that number. It really helps keep the populations in the water
> and not in the garbage can. (Watts 2019)

It took years for her to win her critics over to a model that encourages sustainable
fishing practices. Indeed, she said they thought " 'oh, this little white girl.' After
a year and all the labor, I just blew their mind because they thought that I was
totally full of sh*t" (Watts 2019).

Watt's awareness of her gendered whiteness in the mostly male local fishing community in Hawai'i expresses how her identity shapes her work, and how an intersectional understanding of the gendered and raced dynamics of these relationships evolves over time. These nuances are integral parts of this intersection. Many fishers identify as "local" in Hawai'i, which Jonathan Okamura describes as having a "shared appreciation for the land, the peoples and cultures of the islands" (quoted in Blair 2020). Local identity is often associated with race and ethnicity; it tends to connote descendants of imported plantation laborers, mostly from Asia, who were born in Hawai'i. It may also indicate someone who has lived in Hawai'i since at least high school, and who observes many of the traditional "local" customs. Although white people who are born in Hawai'i sometimes also identify as local, changing demographics and patterns of migration and outmigration are making it more and more difficult to identify who qualifies as local. Ty Kawika Tengan explains that being local means to "have a relationship to place—that is the core issue. It is a commitment to it…to not take the time to understand these histories is really to shirk your responsibility as someone living in these islands" (quoted in Blair 2020). Even though she is white, now that Watts has done the work of integrating herself into the local fisher community and has forged long-standing relationships with "her" fishers, they are more likely to embrace her ideas about resource conservation and its positive long-term effects. As evidenced by the long lines at her farmers' market booth, she has cultivated a successful CSF brand by building loyalty from both fishers and customers at the farmers' markets and through food hubs. That quality ensures that any limitations Watts may have ever thought she might have had are long gone. This kind of hands-on work produces lasting relationships between producers and consumers that contribute to valuing one another's needs and perspectives.

Watts and Rohr break down gendered and racialized barriers in their respective industries to provide locally sourced proteins to people in Hawai'i. In Aotearoa New Zealand, as iwi settlements continue to benefit various iwi in terms of economic development and resources, a series of mandated iwi partnerships in certain agricultural sectors has enabled some Māori to use their cultural practices and traditions surrounding food to change how the private sector relates to sustainable agricultural practices. Fisheries, long harvested sustainably by different iwi, went into a catastrophic decline after colonization led to unrestricted fishing. The 1996 Fisheries Act was implemented unevenly but beginning in 2004, a quota management system was implemented that included a Māori worldview on fisheries, and fish populations have since started to rebound. Much of the original decline stemmed from two issues directly related to colonization. The British government did not acknowledge that Māori conceptualized property in the oceans differently than westerners. This weakened Māori prospects for using their sovereign fisheries rights. Instead, reliance on the British legal concept of the "commons" resulted in overfishing and decimated fisheries through the 1970s and beyond (Hale and Rude 2017). In order to remedy these wrongs for the Māori and the fisheries in question, the Fisheries Settlement Assets were distributed to Mandated Iwi Organizations, and in 2005, an independent reviewer supported expanding this framework to "allow the continued expression of iwi identity and to facilitate their management of their assets as an incidence of ownership" (Castle 2005, cited in Hale and Rude 2017, 70). By January 2015, 98% of fisheries assets had been distributed to iwi through the Mandated Iwi Organizations. The success of the fisheries framework is instructive for other sectors in food and agriculture. Not only are iwi making decisions about their own fisheries, using traditional ecological knowledge to support fish stocks and harvest them sustainably, but they are also feeding their people and profiting within the current capitalist system.

Protein Consumption, Nutrition, and Public Health

The generational impact of healthy food is significant. The basic principles of epigenetics tell us that feeding healthy food to children means that they are more likely to raise their own children the same way (Moss 2025). Decolonizing our palates impacts public and community nutrition and health, as well as our environment. Achieving sustainable community food systems requires eating seasonally, a component of any decolonized diet. Retraining our palates will be an essential step in this process. This means retraining our children to ask for vegetables, or locally grown fish instead of chicken nuggets, and retraining ourselves to not buy mangoes or strawberries when they are out of season. None of this work is easy. Any parent who has watched their child refuse vegetables on the dinner plate can attest to the difficulty of this endeavor. To be sure, re-learning how to cook whole foods from scratch, a process that is essential to feeding families nutritious foods—and that requires time, energy, and the imagination to do so—is difficult as well.

The nutritional value of meat and fish are well-documented. Studies from the National Institute of Health (Pereira and Vicente 2013) and Healthline, which theoretically are not biased toward promoting meat as food (unlike the North

American Meat Institute's website, which touts meat's nutrients as any industry lobby might) extol the virtues of meat-eating as a "superfood for optimal health." Neither of these sources, however, differentiate between factory-farmed meats and pasture-raised, grass-fed beef or farm-raised fish and wild-caught fish. Regenerative agriculture includes animal meat production within its diversified farming practices. Wild-harvested axis deer or feral pigs, for example, offer exceptional nutritional value because they graze in the wild on diverse plants. Harvesting and keeping these protein resources in Hawaiʻi to feed Hawaiʻi's people decreases the need to import meat from elsewhere, which in turn reduces fossil fuel consumption and carbon emissions; reduces the population of invasive species that destroy Native ecosystems; and provides a source of available proteins. Although other forms of protein are certainly available—in beans and vegetables, for example, for those adhering to plant-based diets—these local resources are an excellent dietary option for the large majority of the population, which eats meat on a regular basis.

Meat consumption has been a part of both Native Hawaiian and Māori cultural and culinary practices for centuries. However, raising cattle for human consumption was never meant to become an industry, as is apparent in confined animal feeding operations in the continental United States or in Aotearoa New Zealand. This kind of animal agriculture comes from the colonized histories of both places. Colonizers believed that humans dominating other creatures demonstrated

> cultural superiority. Imposing their livestock system, transforming human-animal relations, and changing the feeding patterns of the natives was a way of 'civilizing' them, which was one of the main objectives of colonization. Thus, food colonialism was not a consequence of the conquest, but an integral part of the imperial project. (Alanes 2022)

The current mode of factory farming, including the dairy industry, reproduces these ongoing colonizing practices.

The colonial legacy of milk production affects Hawaiʻi and Aotearoa New Zealand in different ways, but it is certainly not limited to these two places. Globally, the dairy industry accounts for untold negative environmental consequences, such as polluting waterways, high greenhouse gas and methane emissions, and deforestation (Peterson and Mitloehner 2021). Additionally, it is well-documented that about two-thirds of the world's population are lactose intolerant or malabsorb lactose (Storhaug et al. 2017), including many Indigenous peoples. This fact was willfully ignored by colonizers who pushed milk and dairy consumption on Native peoples in the belief that their breastmilk was inferior to cow milk; in short, they forced Indigenous populations to feed their babies cow milk in an effort to affirm their own standards of decency and grow strong future laborers (Alanes 2022). Aotearoa New Zealand's focus on dairy exports using industrial agricultural practices follows this perspective, but takes the opposite tack of Tait-Jameson's small-scale dairying practices and view of her cows as family members. Tait-Jameson ensures the cows' well-being as well as valuing the relationship between the cows, the humans who raise them, and the quality of their dairy products. Happy cows and goats lead to high-quality milk and associated dairy products. Tait-Jameson in Palmerston North in Aotearoa New Zealand, Bello in Wāhiawa, and the van der Stroom sisters in Waiʻanae (the latter two farms on Oʻahu) can sell their products at a premium because they taste good. This means they can stay in business and continue their animal husbandry (problematic terminology notwithstanding) practices, thereby maintaining the cycle of sustaining their respective animals and environments, as well as their businesses.

Conclusion

If the social media interest in plant-based diets is any indication, then these alternative diets to the factory-farmed, heavily processed, meat-centric western diet certainly have a place in this cultural moment. The women interviewed for this book, however, present other options for meat, fish, and dairy production. In doing so, they demonstrate that small-scale, diversified animal farming operations have a place in island ecosystems with finite resources to maintain biodiversity and rectify environmental damages inflicted by invasive species. Their work exemplifies the ways in which humans and animals are part of a biodiverse ecosystem that mitigates climate impacts, and how supporting locally grown and sourced meat, fish, and dairy products can provide part of a healthy and sustainable diet. Working within industries typically dominated by men, these women propose an alternative way of doing business that relies on valuing the ongoing relationship between humans and animals within finite island ecosystems.

CHAPTER 6

Gifting to Make Connections and Engaging Community to Make Policy

Inherent in a food system is culture, language and identity.
—Lara Shirley (2013)

Gifts of All Kinds

During the research for this project, I learned that gifts create relationships. Gifts from the land stimulate conversation and create an easy entry for talking about sustainable agriculture. As Kimmerer states: "the currency of a gift economy is, at its root, reciprocity" (2013, 28). Sharing food enabled the interviewees and me to find common ground to start talking story. Gifts also foster gratitude—what Kimmerer calls "cultivat[ing] an ethic of fullness" (2013, 111). This exchange of food and ideas, bounty and stories, gifts and laughter showed me the meaning of reciprocity—not in things, but in relationships and abundance. Nancy Red-feather, the long-time director of the Kohala Center on Hawai'i Island, provided additional examples of the gifting economy in the informal food system. Her explanation of the experience of communities growing something in their backyards and exchanging food with their neighbors is not as much about bartering, which involves trading based on some kind of worth or agricultural product value, but rather an informal food system based on gifts of plenty and abundance. Summer Maunakea, an education professor at the University of Hawai'i at Mānoa, who teaches pre-service teachers how to use the garden in their lessons, connects this giving of gifts to women's traditional roles as nurturers, arguing that

> We're supposed to bring life and nurture life and continue to be part of this continuum that allows an ecosystem to continue flourishing and giving life. I think as women, we naturally protect that that cycle. Whether it is birthing children, growing food, we can't get away from it. And I think if you can, it's

just a symptom of a larger social structure or a larger political movement that is taking us away from what we are designed to do. And I would say it comes naturally. (Maunakea 2019)

For Maunakea, these gender roles are rooted in Indigenous cultural values. She sees them as

nourishing the cycle of growth. If you're a teacher, there is that continual growth and feeding of your students. You have to keep their development moving in a healthy direction. If you're a mother, it's in your home. If you're a farmer, it's in growing of your food and nourishing the soil in a way that it's going to continue to provide in a healthy manner. (Maunakea 2019)

Again, this risks an essentialist view of women's roles as mothers, but nurturing here has other connotations, such as nourishing knowledge and soil, which will in turn nourish the people. To do so, we need to support a culture of giving, not just gifts of food, but of health, wellness, power, and of course, life. Sarah Burchard, the chef, food blogger, and farmers' market tour operator, views women's roles through an essentialist lens as well, at the same time as she disagrees that there is any special link between women and this type of work in food and sustainable agriculture. She says:

Women are natural nurturers, right? Caretakers. Anything food-related, service-related and supporting things that are health giving, I feel like it's very, very comfortable for a woman, you know? That's a space we're comfortable in. But I don't think that I'm drawn to this work because I'm a woman, I don't necessarily think that I am more impactful because I'm a woman. (Burchard 2019)

At the same time as she sees a special relationship between women and food due to their traditional roles as nurturers, she does not perceive her own work with food as being linked to her gender identity. Of course, that is her prerogative, but it is an interesting juxtaposition in that she perceives other women as suited for roles in the food system due to their gender identity, but she does not see herself in the same vein. Monica Esquivel also found strength in women's ability to collaborate, listen, and develop relationships. She understood how problematic it was to rely on an essentialist view of gender identity. She stated: "I hate to say it, but I just think we have that inherent part of us that makes us a better fit for this work" (Esquivel 2019). It is difficult to incorporate a critique of essentialism since it is clearly an asset of the women involved in the project. Most of the respondents see it as a part of their power.

Gifting and sharing an abundance of food with neighbors, family, and friends was also seen as a powerful incentive to farm and work in AFNs. Frieda Lotz-Keegan and her mother, Ness Keegan, the permaculture teachers and farmers at PermaDynamics near Whangārei on the North Island of Aotearoa New Zealand, explained that striking a balance between economic survival and sharing abundance with community is difficult, but achievable.

> We have such a strong foundation in being completely regenerative, we're definitely not doing anything we do for money. The basis of why we do something, why we do everything is for the environment and the land. But then also it's not supplemented by something else outside of a job that we have to go to, but actually be able to make it on income off the land. It's another form of inspiration for people so that they really see how we can create human inclusive ecosystems. (Keegan 2020)

Here, we see a distinction between sharing with people and sharing with the land because humans are part of ecosystems and reciprocity is inherent in sustainable agriculture, which of course is rooted in traditional ecological knowledge and Indigenous values. If we take care of the land, it will take care of us.

> And we know and also help food security by creating a surplus, you feed yourself and others. On a community level, exchange level or gift level, whatever. It's still lovely to be able to share food that you've gotten. I think that's having an abundance. Being able to achieve an abundance in a small, relatively small area is inspiring for a lot of a lot of people that come here. And that's lovely. (Keegan 2020)

Keegan expands to discuss the possibility of sharing abundance with others and how that might be instrumental in creating community in one's surrounding area. Trading produce with neighbors, working together to grow different crops so that abundance can be shared, is precisely what a gifting economy is all about.

> That kind of distinction between productivity and production is key because we're so geared towards production. How much land and how much produce can you get out of the land? But productivity is a whole different question. You know, you've got diversity, you've got health of the environment, you've got health of the soils. (Lotz-Keegan 2020)

Being able to make enough money to buy necessary inputs for the farm or make capital investments in equipment is balanced with ensuring that there is enough abundance to gift food to neighbors or, in their case, even visiting students who are taking their permaculture courses. Maintaining this balance also includes caring for the productivity of the soil and the health of the ecosystem. The narrative of abundance can even be overwhelming, as it seems to have been for Trish Allen:

> Coming from the farm where we had so many trees and so many visitors, I thought I needed so many [trees] here in the village. Actually, during the first few years when the trees started producing, I was preserving and making jam and chutneys. And then five years later, I've still got that jam because I can't keep up. So now I just give the fruit away. I supply my sisters, my nieces, my friends, my neighbors. (Allen 2020)

Being able to gift produce and other farm products like value-added jams and chutneys creates food security and community. At Papatūānuku Marae, a woman who was taking a weaving class taught by Hineāmaru Ropati, whom I did not interview in great detail but who did speak to me about her garden, explained that it was her responsibility to share her fruit with others from her orchard, lest it go to waste and not be used to feed people who might need it. Kelly Francis uses her work with Whenua Warrior to gift garden boxes, soil, compost, and seeds to families in marginalized communities in order to work toward food sovereignty in those spaces (2020). She explains that the work has not been without its challenges but said one of her most important points was that there were no profits being made—the gifts of the prepared garden boxes were made possible by a charitable trust structure and donated or free materials. Her ingenuity knows no bounds, as she is able to transform pallets and other discarded items into viable food production spaces.

Strength through and within gender identity was key to some of the respondents. This was an especially valuable when combined with Indigenous cultural values. For example, Ka'iulani Oddom titled the birthing classes at Kōkua Kalihi Valley, "Birthing a Nation"—in other words, raising the *lāhui* (nation). She asserted that she was tired of the deficit model. What makes Kanaka Maoli strong and resilient? In her view: family, culture, and 'āina—"everything you eat every day nourishes the cells of your future generations" (Oddom 2019). During a discussion of generational thinking, Oddom asserted,

> If we're thinking long-term, if we're thinking seven generations, if we're thinking of what kind of world we want, the foundation we want for them to have

> everything we eat, say, and do on a daily basis is nourishing your children and your grandchildren and great-grandchildren. If we look at health from that standpoint, then we have to do a better job. We just have to do a better job. (Oddom 2019)

Her emphasis on the long-term, generational impact of the kinds of foods we eat now is rooted in the genealogical systems-thinking of Kanaka Maoli and Māori.

Indigenous values recognize the long-term implications of our actions. Western colonizers wrote off Indigenous scientific knowledge about sustainable agriculture, among other things, as outdated and "primitive." They discounted it as a valid source of knowledge because it was not based on "modern" scientific evidence. The joke appears to be on western science, though, since the large-scale industrial agriculture model has led to increased inputs, lower returns, and climate and public health crises. Esquivel recognizes that the lost cultural connection between people is "at the bottom of this broken system. The traditional systems, and even in the ones that were forced like the plantation, there was still this economy of sharing. It needs to be restored" (Esquivel 2019). Working through culturally appropriate mechanisms to reinstate certain values like an ethic of sharing, connection, and generative abundance enables entire communities to thrive, not just the privileged few.

Creating Policy Change

Women find many creative ways to push the food systems in Hawai'i and Aotearoa New Zealand to become more sustainable. Their intersectional focus on the current unequal food system is precisely what is driving this transformation forward. Sharing their stories to amplify their voices is an important part of this work. Weaving those stories together enables us to see a bird's-eye view of the network of connections among the work itself and the women doing the work. Much is at stake in controlling the narrative. Following Alcoff's (1991) well-placed hesitance in speaking for others, this work gathers individual stories, so that they may become more powerful through their compilation. I am simply putting the pieces of the puzzle together to provide a more holistic picture of the efforts to fix the food system throughout Oceania. Although I remain uneasy that the project as a whole may be interpreted as me speaking for others, "using" the narratives, or culturally appropriating them, it is critical to center these stories to create a space for political resistance. Following hooks (1984), the point is for the margin to become the center of the discourse surrounding the food system; this entails highlighting shared experiences, not flattening them into the same experiences.

A policy thread runs through the stories of the challenges and opportunities facing those interested in improving Hawai'i's and Aotearoa New Zealand's food systems. I use the word "thread" advisedly here because although it is an unmistakable undercurrent, it would be false to say that current policy supports fixing these food systems. Although some inroads toward that goal have been made through iwi settlements in Aotearoa New Zealand, and there is a mandate to double local food production in Hawai'i, transformative policy remains relatively tenuous. I interviewed several women working in different aspects of policymaking who are pushing the boundaries of food system and sustainable agriculture policy.

Ashley Lukens, one of the founders of the Hawai'i Food Policy Council, came to this work through her dissertation research at the University of Hawai'i at Mānoa, which examined "how identity drove the differentiation of change-making in food justice movements specifically looking at dismantling racism work" (Lukens 2019). She explained that her hypothesis was originally that "white people would typically be drawn toward policy because they didn't have the sort of unconscious or conscious rejection of the state as an ally in making change" (Lukens 2019). This understanding of white privilege is crucial to examining how allyship supports food system transformation at different levels of analysis. For example, there is the actual work done on farms to supply local food to local people. Nevertheless, there are other aspects of the food system that need support from food system experts, such as tracking bills at the legislature and lobbying for sustainable food system-related bills. As she was doing the latter, Lukens saw a need for a Hawai'i Food Policy Council. She discovered that this was an inflection point in the "fastest growing innovation in governance" (Lukens 2019). From there, she focused on debates about genetically modified organisms (GMO) in Hawai'i. Through her research, she learned that GMOs were "probably the most egregious environmental justice issue" (Lukens 2019). Schoolchildren in public schools, especially in rural areas in Hawai'i, are surrounded by miles of experimental GMO cornfields and experience pesticide drift daily. Because Hawai'i has a year-round growing season and is not limited to one crop rotation per year, as farming on the continent is, Bayer Corporation (formerly Monsanto) found that it could run tests three times a year to determine how much pesticide and herbicide its GMO corn could withstand. Prior to the work of Lukens and her fellow activists, there were no buffer zones around schools, and children were exposed to these chemicals every single day. Lukens explained:

I had this very visceral moment where I saw these moms sending their kids to school in communities that were being affected by pesticide drift and my daughter [was] going to Hanalani, this gated community-style school with Hawai'i's wealthiest people. There was this real sense of honor around protecting kids and leveraging the privilege that I had as a *haole* [white or foreign person in Hawai'i, not of Kanaka Maoli descent] with institutional insider access to power brokers. That was the governing conclusion of my dissertation. White people can create relationships that leverage their privilege and their access into institutions. For communities that might have been historically disenfranchised or, in Hawai'i, completely reject the legitimacy of the state, I wondered; can we be that inter-locutor? I had already been recreationally lobbying but I'd never really done it for real before. But I think that's why I was very successful, because there was no roadmap. I didn't know what I didn't know. (Lukens 2019)

Here, Lukens highlights two specific aspects of her food system work: allyship and activism beyond the boundaries of her knowledge and comfort zone. To do this work, one must understand one's privilege to avoid performative allyship; this entails actually doing the work and making sure to lift up the voices of the affected communities themselves by listening and learning and then *doing* the work based on their input. She understood that she was able to foster change through lobbying and Food Policy Council work, yet because she was unfamiliar with the rules of the legislature and the different county councils, she was unafraid of putting herself out there to lobby against a giant corporation.

I quickly took the mom strategy that worked and deployed it in Honolulu, and we started doing these small-scale teas and dinners. I had one presentation, had a professional designer do the slides. It was pretty. It was sexy. It was easy to look at. It took all the data that I had collected over the years, and we just walked people through it in privacy so that they felt comfortable asking questions because again, combat and dissension is not a cultural standard [in Hawai'i]. Specifically for women, I think. And I just knew that if I gave these women enough information and talking points that they could start to counter it. They would go out and spread the same kind of information. I ended up doing 200 of these presentations. (Lukens 2019)

These specific activism strategies are examples of how allyship can work to produce concrete results. Lukens leveraged her policy knowledge from her Food Policy Council work and shared it in intimate settings so that people could ask questions without being afraid to lose face. She mostly spoke to women who were interested in the topic because they were mothers—an example of strategic essentialism at work. The shared experience of motherhood rallied these women to Lukens's anti-GMO cause and ultimately won the day in a very close Maui ballot amendment for a moratorium on GMO crops in 2014.

> For the national audience, which had started to pay attention because of our wins, it was the first time ever that the GMO movement on the mainland was able to understand the environmental justice underpinnings of GMO agriculture because no other case study had so clearly linked the technology with pesticides. (Lukens 2019)

Lukens's experiences are not just performative allyship; she worked with women throughout the state of Hawai'i to change policy and to get laws on the books that would prevent chemical companies from spraying near schools. They won a major victory in Maui County, which eventually spread to the other islands in Hawai'i. Originally, it was not clear whether she included the voices of the affected communities themselves or only focused on certain activists' voices. However, she explains that she went door to door and started having conversations with women. Indeed, she states:

> It was the mother angle that activated them. And it was the fact that they were trying to protect their children. I do think that at least in my work, it was about wanting to do something to protect their children that made women who had previously not been political at all engage in this political resistance movement. "By any means necessary" is as a phrase that pops into my mind. You can see the politicization and food becomes a place where a mom can feel empowered to better or do her best. I would watch women who themselves ate at McDonald's who wanted to learn how to make kale applesauce for their babies. In our lives there are very few life-changing teachable moments, but parenthood is one of them. And that merging consciousness and sense of responsibility for another person and the planet is very powerful. To me, that's a part of what motherhood gives us. (Lukens 2019)

Lukens's activism and leadership generated reprisals from the chemical company representatives and others. A Kaua'i County mayoral candidate at the time openly accused her of using sex to manipulate outcomes and of misappropriating funds. Despite these sexist attacks, the network of female activists protected her and helped her overcome the attacks on her reputation. Hawaiʻi is small and word spread fast, so the state's smallness worked in her favor because people who had been involved in the political resistance to the chemical companies lobbying saw the attacks for what they were: an effort to discredit Lukens's character as a white woman in Hawaiʻi, especially to potential funders. Being a woman in this case was both an advantage and a disadvantage. In the end, Lukens came out of the experience having learned how the political system works, as well as how to navigate the intricacies of networks and relationships to come out unscathed. Although she shared that it seemed like it was a yearlong battle of psychological warfare, she came out stronger for it, as did the anti-pesticide drift policy throughout Hawaiʻi.

Not only does policy change need to happen but, as Daniela Spoto argues, "there is a social norming that needs to change in order to embrace [food system change] as a philosophy" (Spoto 2019). Social norming is a behavior intervention approach often used to promote positive health-related behaviors (Dempsey et al. 2018). Spoto believes that communities need to band together to change food systems, because they cannot accomplish these large-scale changes on their own. Additionally, Amy Brinker, the director of Sustainability Programs at Kamehameha Schools/Bishop Estate, one of the largest landowning trusts in the state of Hawaiʻi with a mission to educate Native Hawaiian children, argues that "what we're doing is not going to last. We're gonna have to turn away from this purely individualistic thing and turn back to these more collectivist cultural practices, Polynesian-style, in this beautiful intersection between food and policy" (Brinker 2019). This collectivist ideal is rooted in many Indigenous cultural values, including those of Hawaiʻi and Aotearoa New Zealand. Working together both in the field/gardens and on policy is critical to achieving any lasting change. Some of the women I interviewed have been working at this for decades. Redfeather was an early proponent of using school gardens as instructional tools and later would create a collective of school gardens, a *hui*, to learn from each other and replicate successful strategies, as well as avoiding pitfalls. She explains her journey to that realization:

> We got another series of grants to create a curriculum map because we realized that the teachers were having a really hard time figuring out how to connect ʻāina-based learning with core curriculum subjects in the classroom. A lot of them aren't gardeners. Sure, if you're a gardener and a teacher and you hear something, that's it. It becomes more obvious to you. But if you're not a gardener, then then you need a map. And so that's what we did for K-8—we aligned these four themes

to all of the core subjects. Common Core Language Arts and mathematics and
next generation science and Hawai'i state health standards and things like that.
(Redfeather 2019)

Working with colleagues at the Kohala Center, Redfeather wrote and distributed
garden education curriculum guides and trained in-service teachers to teach
children through garden projects. These guides are necessary for educators who
do not necessarily have experience with gardening or who might not know how
to react in the face of adversity. From personal experience as a school garden
volunteer for many years, showing up to a garden volunteer day and finding
that feral pigs have dug up and eaten all of the first graders' crops is difficult to
manage, let alone explain, to 30 seven-year-olds. While it is an opportunity to
explain the cycle of life and how different parts of the ecosystem work together,
it is also challenging to console that many kids now that the carrots they have
painstakingly been measuring have vanished.

> The systems that we work with here on this farm, and the systems that
> we're working with the teachers on the school garden curriculum map
> are all ancient systems. People have been using these systems all over the
> world for thousands and thousands of years, so I don't really look at it as
> resistance but more like bringing back some food independence and food
> security that we actually don't have now due to our reliance on globalization.
> (Redfeather 2019)

Redfeather acknowledges the debt that modern agriculture has to traditional
ecological knowledge and is conscious of including Indigenous agricultural practices in school gardens, especially by connecting them to food systems change.
She does not see it as resistance, but a restoration of sustainable agriculture
practices that have already proven their worth since island Indigenous systems
fed communities with no outside inputs for hundreds of years.

> At the legislature, people don't really believe in agriculture anymore. You don't
> see people believing that we can grow our own food or that we can have a
> vibrant agricultural economy that's part of our economy. Because they don't do
> it themselves, they're so far from it. Again, it's that one generation apart. They
> just have not experienced it themselves, nor do they know too many people that
> are doing that. It's just us. As the years go on, I think this is getting worse rather
> than better. (Redfeather 2019)

This passage echoes some other Hawai'i-based narratives about how the descendants of plantation laborers, who are now entrenched in educational institutions, want to have nothing to do with the kind of agriculture their parents experienced—backbreaking, dawn-to-dusk, exploitative plantation labor. They remember their parents working in the sugar cane or pineapple fields for low pay and cannot fathom anyone wanting to support agriculture as a profession. I remember going with several teachers to speak to the principal at my children's high school to ask her if we could start an afterschool volunteer garden club for interested students. She looked at us blankly and asked us "why?" Redfeather echoes this resistance to agricultural education from Department of Education administrators as well.

> We're just trying to give them an appreciation for where their food comes from, how to take care of the land, and what is good stewardship. Environmental education was dropped from the school system in 1999, so just kind of reinstituting environmental education. It's a big, broad kind of area but then they would all grow up knowing that they could put a garden or small orchard in their backyard if they wanted to and also know the value of the local food. They're going to be consumers for as long as they live here, and it would give them all a chance to really understand how precious this food is that comes from Hawai'i. (Redfeather 2019)

Redfeather's appreciation for the importance of traditional ecological knowledge as well as raising children's awareness of local food and its sources is critical in her policy advocacy. She understands the important role of education policy in supporting these systems and spent decades pushing for additional awareness at the levels of the schools, the Department of Education, and the Hawai'i State Legislature. Although she has been successful, she is the first to admit that there is more work to be done, and in some cases, undone.

Because there is little emphasis on the nonprofit sector to address social and environmental problems, much of the focus in Aotearoa New Zealand depends on business to solve problems. As Tennant et al. (2008) argue, "the influence of the neo-liberal doctrines had profound implications for the nonprofit sector in this most recent period of its history" (32). There is not a long history of relying on nonprofit organizations to service the needs of society, especially surrounding environmental and sustainability issues. Most nonprofit organizations in Aotearoa New Zealand employ no staff at all (Tennant et al. 2008). For much of its history, after colonization, volunteerism was predicated on patriotism and religion, both sentiments that have declined precipitously in the past few decades. Within this landscape, however, several of the organizations discussed in this book, as well as certain Māori organizations, certainly qualify as nonprofit organizations, even if they do not necessarily fit with the western (read: accepted and mostly US-centric) model of nonprofit organizations, which provides tax-exempt status to organizations working for the common public good. In fact, in Aotearoa New Zealand, as of this writing there is no single accepted definition of nonprofit status. This divergence does not imply that one type of response to problems surrounding food systems is better than others, but simply that there are a variety of ways to address them. This book examines those responses through the voices of the women doing the work on the ground and in the ground—cultivating the land, the people, and community so that each component thrives.

Policy work, whether at the individual or organizational level, is also key to several of the interviewees in Aotearoa New Zealand. Jenny Lux, the owner operator of Lux Organics in Rotorua, explained that it was important to be involved in policy conversations in her community to ensure representation for small farms and marae to be able to "sell organic without too many barriers. It's a bit of an area of debate, because there's always conflict between big organic and small" (Lux 2020). Whether this involvement is based on running a small agricultural business or trying to work within the settlement legislation, the mandated power-sharing agreement puts "iwi in a really strong position for future development" (Francis 2020). In fact, Kelly Francis speculated that this policy structure would enable iwi to become as powerful as the government because resolutions to many issues facing Land Back movements were imminent all-around Aotearoa New Zealand. She explained that legal strategies used by iwi to fight the colonial land grab were finally coming to fruition, especially at Ihumātao Village, where she lives (Francis 2020). Yet, a passing comment by Kate Cherrington after I had put away my recording device is instructive here. She claimed that the country was at a political and cultural moment of reckoning and that although the prime minister at the time, Jacinda Ardern, was a strong leader, the Māori situation was really just "more of the same" (Cherrington 2020). She claims that it is up to Māori iwi to push for change, and she sees the tribal structure as an integral part of that process. I would also argue that the existence of marae as a dedicated space for civic and community engagement is a driving force in this journey.

Community Engagement

Because food is instrumental in bringing people together, many respondents saw it as a critical tool for engaging community, as with Koethe's networks of women farmers, Ladrig's farmer field trips to see how others are dealing with specific agricultural problems, Morgan-Bernal and Huff's engagement of thousands of schoolchildren through school gardens under the auspices of the Hawai'i Department of Education, or Oddom's community work days at Kōkua Kalihi Valley to engage Micronesian and Pasifika women to grow culturally appropriate foods that they can then share during cooking demonstrations at the clinic. Food draws people in and encourages them to stay. Participants are more likely to engage in conversation about its importance and how we can find ways to get good local food to families and communities if it is culturally appropriate, healthy, and tasty. Sometimes, these conversations are the initial touchpoint for women's voices to bubble up from marginalized spaces, all the way to the halls of power. For example, Spoto says she often feels patronized at the legislature: "women's voices are not as valued in that building. The policy side of things garners a lot of business interests and those are male-dominated. Those voices tend to just get a lot more airtime" (Spoto 2019). When she was a part of the Hawai'i Farmer's Union, Ladrig felt that she didn't know enough to have a strong voice and didn't feel like she was supported enough. When another woman voiced her opinion, other union members derided her for being "too bossy," and Ladrig did not want to follow in her footsteps. It left her feeling "like a girl, not a woman" (Ladrig 2019), and she didn't want to participate in promoting internal conflict. As negative as these experiences were, they cannot be ignored. It is difficult to organize others or to be a leader in a space that is hostile toward women. The respondents in this book have consistently shown up and done the work. They have carved out spaces where there had previously been none, and they have seen that the moment to make changes is now. Spoto says "for all intents and purposes, we should be the leaders, because if we can't figure it out for ourselves in terms of the stage of life for the climate crisis and potential shipping disruptions, who can? We can figure out how to feed ourselves and do it healthily" (Spoto 2019). The key issue here is that climate change and the global COVID-19 pandemic are pushing us to reframe our ideas about the food system, especially in island ecosystems. Spoto and many others in this study have stepped in to fill the void, because no one else was poised to do so.

Leadership takes many forms, though. Spoto says she reframed her role to be more of a content-area expert, rather than a leader herself. However, without her expertise, other leaders could not make their voices heard, especially if they weren't provided with the right evidence. When asked how she saw her leadership around food system issues, she answered that she saw herself as more of a facilitator than a leader. Many participants echoed this sense. Their conception of leadership was not ego-driven or competitive. Rather, it focused on collaboration, mentoring, and grassroots activism—all of which provide opportunities for everyone to shine. Although several women ascribed this leadership style to a more feminine approach to organizing, I am reluctant to reiterate those sentiments. Rather, it seems like collaborative leadership is more prevalent in organizations that grow from grassroots community activism. For example, if there is information about grant opportunities, the members of the Good Food Alliance will try to figure out how to use it to benefit multiple partners in the organization, rather than hoarding the information and opportunity for themselves and/or their own organization in order to win the competitive grant process. This demonstrates the benefits of decentralized knowledge to regionalizing the food system and working from the ground up (sometimes, quite literally) to accomplish certain goals.

The Kohala Center on Hawai'i Island was built on a collaborative organizational culture. Cole explained that "women have the inclination, the skill set, and to some extent the will, to take time to sit in these meetings" (Cole 2019). And while that can be beneficial in several ways, part of it is problematic because it ties into the notion that women can and should "have it all," which is really shorthand for women should "do it all." Leaning in is overrated and exhausting if one does not have help in the home to care for children or the house. Joleen Oshiro argues that women's flexibility is what puts them front and center in food system transformation:

> I think that when you're dealing with something that's transforming and growing and changing, women are especially pivotal in something like that because our world has gotten a lot grayer. I think we multi-task, and we juggle, and we are flexible because we have to be, because just in our own personal lives, we're probably wearing three or five hats at any given time. And by the time we add in the work, because women have to work since there are not many who can stay home and raise kids, it requires a lot of flexibility, a lot of thinking out of the box. Now, there's a lot of space right now for people to meet to create something that will work. I mean, it really is a movement, right? (Oshiro 2019)

Oshiro rightly points out that food system change has to be a collective movement and has to start with community input. In her work, she sees that it is mostly women doing this work, and finding creative ways to juggle a multitude of tasks to make change happen. But this is not easy work.

Why is it that this labor falls to women? Because it includes food? Because it includes nourishment? Because those tasks are traditionally associated with women? The kitchen can also be a place of resistance, revolution, and creativity. For example, the seminal feminist text entitled *This Bridge Called My Back* was originally published by Kitchen Table: Women of Color Press. The name of the publishing company was no accident. Shared experiences of marginalization by feminist academics of color galvanized them to start their own publishing company to change what counted as academic writing. The same goes for the ongoing food system revolution. Again, if this work is unpaid or underpaid, who has access to becoming involved becomes problematic. Given the high cost of living in Hawai'i, for example, people working multiple jobs to make ends meet are unlikely to be able to attend Food Policy Council meetings or anti-GMO rallies, or go down to the legislature to lobby for school lunch reform. This privileges certain viewpoints, and while we would like to think that those perspectives benefit everyone, this kind of short-sighted behavior can exacerbate tensions between communities and increase problems within marginalized communities.

Because food system transformation work is underpaid or even unpaid, and since women are the ones stepping up to do it, the food system is reproducing the structural inequality found in so many other gendered spaces. As Gearon argues, "women's work is the original subsidy for capitalism" (2021). The work of the Good Food Alliance is unpaid. The women who come to the meetings are paid in their other capacities, and they attend Zoom meetings from their islands as part of their duties, but the networking aspect of the organization, which is vital to its continued success, is not specifically remunerated. One of the major concerns with this unpaid labor is that it does not ascribe a monetary value to the work, even though the work is vital to community health and well-being. An additional issue is that it tends to continually shift the focus back toward per-sonal responsibility and individual consumer choices, instead of focusing on the organizational dynamics of systems-thinking and structural inequalities. Lukens asserts that the alternative food movement has "to its peril, relied too heavily on individual action. [Furthermore,] there is a culture of silence in Hawai'i. It's like an underbelly, a shadow side of the food movement here. There's a lot of unspoken, problematic sexism" (Lukens 2019). Given her academic work on whiteness and privilege in grassroots movements in a settler colonial space, it is possible that Lukens would be likely to recognize sexism as it was happening. Yet, both Rohr and Watts (the "meat" and "fish ladies" respectively, as they call themselves), also encountered sexism in their work in industries that tend to be extremely male-dominated. For example, when Esquivel seemed to say that she felt like an imposter, she found solace in the support network of the Good Food Alliance. The notion of supporting each other is tied to supporting local food and sustainable agriculture and food system actors. It's a network of mutual aid that enables women to thrive. Farmers are able to increase production, families can eat healthier, and communities flourish. This exemplifies the strengths perspective that Maunakea and Higa highlighted in their narratives. If we look to what communities are doing right, even in the face of what seem like insurmountable odds, like poverty driven by ongoing neocolonial practices, we can see that healing communities is within reach. Using a systems-perspective adds complexity to thinking about food. Williams explains that women have a "different perspective and angle on systems. This is really critical and something that is making a big difference" (Williams 2019). During her education, she explains she was reluctant to focus on one single thing and realized that sustainability is made up of a variety of connected sectors and factors. Focusing narrowly on one aspect of the food system is precisely what has led us to a broken food system. Systems-thinking enables us to analyze different aspects of the food system to see how they interact and how they can be strengthened to benefit the whole.

In a seminal essay originally published in 1989, and reprinted hundreds of times, Wendell Berry explained that eating is an agricultural act (2009). Pollan moved that concept toward the political (2006), saying that we make political choices three times a day, by deciding what kinds of food we eat at every meal. This is all true, of course, but the spirit of "voting with your fork" is simply not enough to foster wholesale food system change because it relies on individuals to make a difference, when systemic solutions are needed as well. On a smaller scale, people who don't do this work for a living often do not think of the garden and foodways a place of, or for, politics. But are they? What is politics in this sense? Is the garden devoid of politics? Is the kitchen? The cafeteria? I'd argue that they do indeed constitute political spaces, but perhaps not in the sense of the kind of politics we tend to associate with the public sphere. Are we in the garden as consumers? Maybe. Are we in the garden as creators? Yes. Are we in the garden as citizens? Also, yes. For example, as Sarah Smuts-Kennedy argues "we are co-sharing problem solving and innovation. We love knowing what everyone is doing, so we feel deeply connected. Farming can be a very lonely thing, but urban farmers are generally quite social people" (Smuts-Kennedy 2020). Her intent is to avoid separating the commons from the commons, to avoid building fences to separate people. This attitude of willingness to share and to take a risk on community involvement is integral to maintaining relationships within community. She acknowledges that the land is Māori, so it is important to look to their guidance prior to starting any new projects. She wants to include land and spiritual acknowledgments in the For the Love of Bees projects to honor their ancestors and Māori ancestral knowledge, much as Jacqui Forbes, Hineāmaru Ropati, Pounamu Skelton, and Kate Cherrington all mentioned was a central element in any respectful food system transformation. While Smuts-Kennedy is Pākehā, she is trying to use food system projects in an urban area like Auckland to get people talking about Māori values. Like Skelton, she sees gardens, whether urban or rural, as places where people come to get nourishment and even sisterhood. Skelton told me that she encourages people to talk, especially women, to know that their voice matters: "In Māoridom, men speak, and women sing. That's always been big" (Skelton 2020). Like Smuts-Kennedy, she wants to hear their voices, because what they have to say is important. It is essential for community engagement to reflect everyone's voice, especially voices that have traditionally been marginalized. Many of the women interviewed for this project recognized the value of not just hearing women's voices, but really listening to what they have to say. Their experiences growing or consuming food show that making these connections with others is central to one's well-being—and all the more so if it is being done with hands turned to the soil, together.

Stories as Seeds of Change

The relational aspect of this project drives the connections among participants' stories. We can think of it as a garden, which requires patience and observation, as well as trial and error. The stories are seeds. Some will grow and blossom into larger ideas and innovations, while others might not succeed or take hold. But as a whole, a garden teaches as much as it provides food, joy, and transformation. The women doing this work embody the combination of strength and flexibility of women the world over. They have applied their skills specifically to the food system in innovative ways to find a more sustainable way to feed ourselves and our communities. The relationships among, and the stories of the producers, consumers, food writers, public health advocates, grant writers, cooperative managers, farmers' market vendors and managers, farm-to-school activists and educators, policy advocates, cafeteria managers, CSA managers, food pantry coordinators, sustainability planners, and chefs create the framework for implementing a better food system. These connections create pathways for exchanging ideas, food, networks, and platforms.

Working together, the women interviewed often overlap and learn from each other so as not to have to reinvent the wheel. If a project works on one island, it can be shared and replicated on other islands. If there are certain challenges to specific projects, they can be identified to prevent them from occurring again, or someone who had a similar experience elsewhere might have an idea for how to mitigate the problem. This potential for exchange creates possibilities. Almost all the women interviewed for this project identified their own roles as being connectors or said they participated in spaces of exchange where the connectors were all women. Amy Brinker, the Sustainability Coordinator for Kamehameha Schools, linked this role to women being what she called "systems-thinkers" (Brinker 2019). Although I initially bristled at the essentialist implications of ascribing this label to women, I soon realized that the reason systems-thinking is prevalent among women is because of the incredible amount of multitasking they must do in order to succeed. Brinker claims that this "level of complexity requires holding a lot of different things simultaneously in our head. As we think of solving food systems, we inherently have to address other things like gender relations. It's an interesting dynamic" (Brinker 2019). Finding ways to promote this systems-thinking is like moving around different pieces of a puzzle together until they fit properly. Tina Tamai's Good Food Alliance, as a network of networks, and Harmonee Williams' role as the director of Sustʻāinable Molokaʻi both exemplify these connections in different ways. Tamai focuses on policy, education, and sharing information among members of the alliance. Williams's organization connects the farmers with eaters and tries to figure out what works for both sides (Williams 2019). Williams sees this as an extension of the emotional labor women traditionally do in families— bringing family members together to work out differences or to celebrate together for holidays, all of which requires planning and coordination.

On a larger scale, this labor creates community in places where there might not have been any. In some ways, this embodies the restoration of ancestral abundance. Samson sees an important cultural component in this work. She says a lot of women do this work because their parents became disengaged and lost their connection to their culture, their land, and their communities. However, she asserts that women invest heavily in this work because they don't want to sacrifice their family's health. While again, this places the burden of care on women, it is integral to many of their lives. The reality for most heterosexual relationships is that partnerships are not necessarily co-equal, with each spouse/partner doing half the work. Yet, relying on an understanding of Indigenous cosmology, Oddom explains the value of creating a space for women to thrive no matter their respective family situations. She looks into the past and the future at the same time when she says:

It's important that the land be healthy. That lets people be healthy and our community be healthy. And so that's really important to me. I make my decisions on what's best for the community, not what's best for myself. Up in the valley where I started is Haumea. That's our legends. And our stories tell us that she resided there. For women to *be*...There are some really great men, don't get me wrong, but *it's a woman's world up there. We thrive there* (emphasis added). Food has traditionally been a woman's area in a home economics and dietetics sense. I mean, that's been a woman's world. I think we just transition easily because women are great fighters. I think we're going to fight for things that are important to our children and our grandchildren and so on. We're going to fight for these things because we know the job. (Oddom 2019)

Oddom sees the food system as a space of resistance, both through nutrition and feeding people, as well as gardening and producing crops for community. She also roots the work in past resistance. She says women fight for what they want, because they understand the implications of doing nothing, which has been the status quo for the past few generations.

Rangimārie Mules explains that this new generation of feminism exists all across Māoridom, and the fact that Māori are "allowed to express [their] culture how it's meant to be expressed without a colonial rhetoric means that [they can] finally just *be* without having to call it cultural revitalization" (Mules 2020). Unlike in previous generations, Māori can practice their culture in the open without fear of retribution; this freedom to restore whakapapa and ancestral abundance empowers young female leaders. They can use their platforms to focus on food systems, without having to stop each time and re-explain the importance of Māori culture to this movement. Mules's vision of female leadership within food systems is that

everyone has to eat, drink, and have shelter. These are a few basic human needs that highlight female leadership. We need structural and systemic change in how we value female leadership. It should be adaptive to whatever the context is at the time, but it's an all-around invitational leadership style where you invite people into different spaces, and you encourage capacity or confidence built in others. (Mules 2020)

Similarly, Jacqui Forbes asserts that:

We put our head down. For this past project, we made the system more efficient. We just did it. And I feel like sometimes that attitude is something that the men don't have necessarily. They are maybe looking for the recognition, whereas the women are just going to do it and not talk about it (Forbes 2020).

Forbes's work embodies Juanita Sundberg's (2017) FPE-inspired call to highlight women as agents of environmental change. Forbes and her colleagues are putting their heads down and doing the work, without discussing it at length beforehand. Forbes valued this type of behavior in her team and fostered the collective mindset required to accomplish their goals.

> That's how important it is, the caring for the well-being and mana of the people. We always try to look for the space where both are being upheld. I think it's definitely that the nurture and care, looking after people and working for the common good principles that come through and guide us. It's all about the service to others. You do that work because you can contribute the most there. (Forbes 2020)

In essence, Forbes argues that men look for recognition, but women do the actual work. For example, Hilary Bowen, the co-owner of The Front Room Café in Waikanae Beach, near Wellington was reluctant to take any credit for her work as a leader in farm-to-table dining, saying that she is "just a cook" (2020). She didn't see herself as being groundbreaking, and just did the work because it was her job, not for any higher systems-changing or altruistic purpose. Yet the result is that the restaurant is well-known on the Kapiti Coast for its locally sourced and sustainable ingredients. Only a few of the interviewees compared men's and women's attitudes toward food system work this concretely. Skelton was another Hua Parakore instructor who was clear on the gendered attitudes toward work. She said that

> a majority of my students are women, like 90%. Men might start, but they don't finish often. They just don't finish. They kinda come but don't stay, mostly because women can work together because they know there's something bigger at stake. Women are really strong and resilient and growing their children to be that as well because you can do this job with small children. I think because we have a Māori *kaupapa* [a philosophy or set of principles]. We embrace the whole family. We embrace the farmer, encourage our children to come home. (Skelton 2020)

Women can work together, she argues, because they can look at the larger picture from a systems-oriented perspective and because they understand the implications of learning how to grow food in sustainable ways—it will feed their families healthy food, and often for much cheaper costs (although it definitely will be more time intensive) than going to the supermarket or the fish-and-chip shop.

The cultural, political, environmental, health, and community implications of food systems transformation are colossal. Jenny Lux argues that women's ability to forge social connections is a driving force behind change. She places the argument in a larger context while also questioning her own logic:

> if the world were run by women, we'd be looking after the environment better because we just have more care for the earth. I don't know if that's really true. But maybe if we hadn't had such a patriarchy for so many centuries, we would be in a better situation. Who knows to begin with? (Lux 2020)

Skelton explains that women "hold the future inside of them. I think women generally live much more peacefully than men. We're in that realm all the time. We're growing food, so it's nurturing. It's peaceful. You do these tasks because you want to take care of the plants" (Skelton 2020). Although this can certainly be labeled essentialist thinking, it also reflects Lux's and Skelton's view that women are empathetic, so they are able to form relationships with each other and with nature based on mutual trust and respect. If we respect the land and nourish it, in turn, it will nourish us. Angela Clifford explicitly mentioned essentialism in her narrative, and explained her view this way:

> I get nervous about essentialism. The idea that we are who we are because we are a gender, because the extrapolation goes to a not very nice place. But I definitely do think those aspects of some of this work that is perhaps more appropriate for how women have been socialized as part of society. That includes a lack of ego. Because you have to be all about the collaborative power and about that connection about creating networks and being an enabler or a connector. And you can't do that work if you want to lead alone or from the front or have the recognition solely for you, that just doesn't work. I think often women are better suited to that style of leadership at things. I think there's something to be said about women's connection to the earth. I mean, I find it personally a very meaningful connection. So perhaps it has something to do with it as well. That sort of groundedness, empathy, ability to see other people's perspectives. Patience. (Clifford 2020)

That ability to connect and to empathize is clearly *not* intrinsic in *all* women. To assert that it is leads us to uncomfortable generalizations I am very keen to avoid. That said, in reflecting on the narratives for this research, discussion of collaboration, systems-thinking, long-term visions, and respect for land—all stemming from Indigenous cultural values—came up again and again. These mesh well with individuals and organizations that prize sharing knowledge and disseminating information among group members. As Clifford says, that kind of work is not feasible if one is looking for individual recognition.

Collaborative organizations like the Good Food Alliance are safe spaces where leaders can develop skills to forge partnerships within the food system. Williams viewed the value of collaboration and working together as evident, especially so that no one wastes time replicating work unnecessarily, and being able to do so much more if everyone is working together toward the same goal. She called this a "very feminine perspective" (Williams 2019). Others saw female-led spaces as lacking ego, valuing each other's work, and lifting up each other's successes. Frankie Koethe's development of the women's farmers network through the O'ahu Natural Resources Defense Council is a concrete example of these core values. The idea is to share information among the network of female farmers. To this end, she organizes field trips to different female-led farms on the different islands, started a Facebook group, and promotes different projects through social media posts. These networking ideas create small communities or knowledge hubs around sustainable local food production and consumption.

Communities like these are generated intentionally, and are unlikely to spring up out of nowhere, if only due to the geographic barriers of island life. Although the ocean does connect us, it also makes it more difficult to travel—especially, as we now know, during a pandemic. Many of these projects had to adjust their goals, ways of interacting with each other, and their intended beneficiaries. Yet the idea that community has a voice in determining their food system has remained intact. Tamai and Oddom, for example, are adamant that they support communities working to shape their own food systems, because communities know their own needs best (Tamai 2019; Oddom 2019). Tamai sees this work as identifying resources to support place-based food systems to form one big network composed of "intersecting mini-networks" (Tamai 2019). This focus on interconnectivity is also present in Morgan-Bernal's, Redfeather's, Huff's, and Cole's work. They were all at one point part of Tamai's Good Food Alliance and implemented various iterations of farm-to-school programs on different islands. They focus on communication and appear to find that easier to achieve among like-minded women. This is not to say that they exclude men from their work, but rather that their successes have largely come from working together with other women in food system spaces. Redfeather says that women "have more of a sense of wanting to nurture the earth themselves and their families and communities for whatever reason, probably things that they learned through their families and through life" (Redfeather 2019). Maunakea, like Oddom, roots that nurturing aspect through growing food with the energy of Haumea, the goddess of fertility and birth in Kanaka Maoli creation stories, and explains that it grows life and creates a foundation for home.

The idea of home is based in a variety of conceptions of mothering throughout these narratives. Judd argues that the mother is the "original food provider, since women are often in charge of the kitchen at home" (Judd 2019). For Judd, feeding children is an inherent part of raising children, and for Samson, that love is demonstrated through growing, cooking, and gifting food to and for others. How we love our children and care for each other is the same way we should be taking care of plants, she says (Samson 2020). Similarly, Sana equates growing food with growing good people. She says growing food is all "practice to be a good person: to love, to respect, and the willingness to learn and to work" (Sana 2019). Cooking for people and families, which tends to fall mostly to women, though not always of course, is also a part of loving and growing healthy people. Dana Shapiro explains that she usually makes dinner in her household. In addition to cooking, she thinks about what to prepare, shops for the ingredients, and then does the cooking. She asserts that this is how she was brought up, and that it is part of her cultural upbringing. As much as we would like to resist traditional gender roles, the reality is that many women continue to carry the mental load for feeding families. What is important to remember here is the importance of food to families: it is present during family meals, during celebrations, during holidays, to mark special occasions, to connect people. Ladrig associates her grandmother's house with food, as many of us might, and shares that food makes those memories more tangible (Ladrig 2019). Sullivan shares that the origin of her interest in food and foodways is "very personal, and is about us both as consumers, but also as a family. These are what makes us actors, what gives us agency. Food and agriculture are a space that is generative of community well-being" (Sullivan 2019). Relating food and family to agency highlights the gendered aspects of the food system at the micro-level, its implications for the macro-level, and all the spaces in between.

The women interviewed for this book are among the most important change agents in the food system space in Hawai'i and Aotearoa New Zealand. Their networking efforts with each other and willingness to reach out to various groups and individuals doing similar work was my most useful resource in this project. This demonstrates that their shared and collaborative leadership model means that everyone benefits. When there is no emphasis on ego or seeking credit for accomplishments, the respondents agreed that they were happy to put their heads down and do the work. This is problematic to a certain degree because it adds an additional burden to women's work. This work occurs in gendered, raced, classed, and colonized spaces, but the fact that the work is proceeding and that food systems are being reevaluated is a positive step for all communities.

Redefining Success

Western society defines success through wealth and tends to penalize those who do not fit into the accepted capitalist mold. Kaʻiulani Oddom refuses to judge the success of Kōkua Kalihi Valley's work in capitalist terms. She asserts that

> if you were to judge us just by making money, we wouldn't be a great success. But if you're to judge us by getting fresh fruits and vegetables into the community, having a place to come where people know there's good food for our café hours, people just come to have good conversations and laugh and talk and to tell their story, it's a tremendous success. (2019)

This undoing of the definition of success is only part of the picture, though. Oddom goes on to describe what outsiders think of her community:

> This really allowed us to look into our community and look for all of the positives and the strengths of our communities. People hear about police here; they think about gangs and violence and war. Everybody has a low socioeconomic status. Yet, we have great results in our community. Because one of the things that drives us all together is food. (Oddom 2019)

Kōkua Kalihi Valley has figured out how to incorporate Indigenous cultural values into their food and education programs, linking food with ʻāina, as well as encouraging other cultural events to foster intercultural understanding and appreciation. They call their "CSA boxes CS ʻai using cultural structures" (2019) since ʻai means to eat in ʻŌlelo Hawaiʻi. In addition,

> One of the things we kept hearing from everybody was that they don't have the time to cook and prepare the stuff, so we cooked and prepared three sets and they can take it home and then just throw it in on the stove or make patties with it or whatever they want to do. That's one way that I see us as community supported agriculture. And then we do value added. We also do a lot of community events.

We have what's called an 'Ohana Health Program. I take third to fifth graders over a year, their families have to commit to come in twice a month and we cook with them every other month. We set up nine stations around here and their parents learn to cook. I really feel like kids aren't growing up learning how to cook. They need to learn how to cook. We just do cultural things with them. We do hikes with them. We do mommy classes with them. We just we have family dinners once every other month where we have some type of health topics, but culturally or from a more global setting. They have to come to the school, but they get a dinner. (Oddom 2019)

Lack of access to healthy and fresh food being only one indicator of poverty in Hawai'i, lack of Indigenous knowledge is also part of the problem. Kaui Sana argues that wealth can also be measured in the knowledge found in traditional Indigenous families. She asks, however, "how do you amplify that? How do you support that? And how do you innovate around that" (2019)? These questions lead us to focus on transforming the food system and valuing women's roles in that transformation. Indeed, Betsy Cole (2019) stated that "working in a capitalist context" makes reviving rural incomes nonviable. The American success story is founded on the kind of success that translates to monetary wealth. But rural and island lives do not necessarily follow that model—being rich in produce and community relationships is, for many respondents, a more important determinant of wealth than money. Mules (2020) agrees with Cole's assessment when she says that while we may come from rural backgrounds that are often marginalized and underserved, we do not necessarily want to serve the rich, but we need to influence the rich and powerful so that we can change things. She claims that the way to do this is "to be flexible, so that empathy and compassion lead our negotiations" (Mules 2020). For some that might look different than for others. For example, Frieda Lotz-Keegan and Ness Keegan at PermaDynamics both asserted that demonstrating success by having an economically viable regenerative agriculture operation is only one way to demonstrate that success. Success is not necessarily measured by making a lot of money, but by being self-sustaining and using sustainable agricultural practices. Jacqui Forbes, who understands that we live in a capitalist system that privileges monetary gain no matter how modest, offered yet another, completely different definition of success:

Success comes from giving and sharing, rather than how much you can acquire for yourself. We point out that the current paradigms places money in GDP and economic growth. It's the gods to bow down to. Our Māori paradigm is about interconnectedness and relationships and reciprocal relationships. So you give, you receive, you give and you receive. But you might say that an Indigenous value is your mana and how much you can give away and how much you can care for others. Other paradigms like the current one, wherein your prestige is how much can you get? How much can you acquire and have for yourself? (Forbes 2020)

Gifting, offering, and sharing—often in the form of food—constitute and build relationships. Forbes's description of how people alternate between giving and receiving shows the mutable characteristics of these relationships. She outlines that process as one that defines success. She also decries the focus on amassing wealth or status in the western conception of achievement.

The whole way of thinking is broken too. If we can put more [emphasis on] look[ing] after people, more love, more kindness, more respect, more consider-ation, thoughtfulness, equality, justice and to add these to the paradigm and in our world, then I think it's much easier. (Forbes 2020)

Forbes contextualizes success in terms of her Māori culture and asserts that it should have a wider application to the larger society. And again, monetary gain has nothing do with her definition of success. Similarly, Skelton focused on the ability to pass on knowledge as key to success (Skelton 2020) due to her Māori upbringing steeped in cultural traditions.

Throughout the interviews, appreciating Māori cultural values appeared to be generational. Whereas Forbes and Skelton were raised to appreciate their heritage, other respondents described other paths to (re)discovering their Māori heritage. Cherrington was raised

with gardens and foraging for food and fishing for eels as a part of daily life and in this place. But growing up in the 70s and 80s through the 90s, the signal of your wealth was whether you could go to the supermarket and buy the bread that's sliced. I remember thinking "we'll know when we've arrived because we can shop at the flash supermarket." Because that's what we were programmed to believe, that if you can move away from the homemade, that's the signal of wealth. (Cherrington 2020)

Cherrington returned to her Māori way of thinking by measuring wealth as the ability to care for others and help Māori families tie themselves back to the land. In doing so, they find they can nourish themselves and their communities. Lux agreed, from a Pākehā perspective, that doing something to feed people and to inspire people to garden, even on a small scale, is success. This is especially true if the motivation is not monetary gain, but

> putting good energy out there and getting it back. Money's important, but it's just a form of energy. And usually, the best payment is an appreciative customer or family that says they can't do without your wonderful food. There is an abundance of opportunity for everyone. If we want to feed our communities from local businesses, then we need to set up a system where we can have an abundant mindset and share with each other. It's all about ethics, isn't it? (Lux 2020)

This reflects an asset mindset that values empathy and cooperation, rather than a competitive mindset that would encourage undercutting one's business rival. This view does reflect a certain privilege of course, because without money, it's difficult to pay bills, keep the lights on, put gas in one's car, or even maintain farm equipment.

Thinking beyond short-term profits and understanding how alternative food networks can lead to food system restoration is a critical component of change. Kay Baxter, a woman whom other interviewees called the "grand dame of seed saving" in Aotearoa New Zealand, sees saving seeds as "women's work in the best way" (Baxter 2020). However, Baxter's view is decidedly capitalist. She argues that without assigning a monetary value to seeds, they are not prized or respected within the economy. Without ascribing this monetary importance to seeds, she argues that they will simply disappear. She told me that:

> There was a time that saving seeds was the most important job in any village because if it wasn't done well, people would starve. Working with seeds was women's work. I feel like it's my job and responsibility to the next generation. I feel lucky to be able to do it.
>
> Seeds have been our teacher in many ways. They've led the journey. People that are working in this field have a strong connectedness to the world around them and a strong intuitive link like that requires some kind of connection and empathy for life around us to have the confidence and get the positive feedback to keep doing this kind of work. So it's probably a set of people with high levels of connection to the natural world and who have strong empathy for life around them, which is mostly women. (Baxter 2020)

Baxter's narrative reveals the contradiction of capitalism with generational thinking and looking toward the long-term future. It shows that she embraces what is fundamentally an extractive economic model. This conflict was present in most of the narratives, but Baxter was the only one who really spelled it out. Kelly Francis explained that while she while she diverged with Baxter on whether food and seeds should be free to everyone, she respected her long-time efforts with saving seeds (2020). Indeed, as Hutchings argues: "saving seed, essential to our survival, is a task that has often been undertaken by women" (2015, 39). Baxter follows this tradition, even though she is Pākehā, in order to share and cultivate bounty and to propagate heirloom varieties of plants and trees. Baxter's view is that she has chosen this kind of low-consumption lifestyle and thus has learned to make do with less, even while growing food in abundance (Baxter 2020). While she may not drive a flashy car or wear fancy clothes, her ability to feed her family and community means that she is privileged to have the land to be able to do so. By extension, this requires supporting small farmers with regional distribution and food hub systems so that their food can get into the hands of people who don't have access to food-growing spaces.

Climate Change Resilience

Climate change resilience drives many of the necessary changes to the global industrial food system. Decentralizing this system will create a more just and sustainable food system. Respondents in Hawai'i and Aotearoa New Zealand shared their climate concerns and many of them contextualized their work within the climate crisis. Some had studied the issue at university, others had come to it through professional training, and others through activism. Most focused on shifting our values paradigm to focus less on consumption and on measuring GDP through money passing through the economy, whether for good or bad purposes, because they viewed the capitalist accumulation system as inherently problematic. While none of the respondents mentioned the Genuine Progress Indicator, which includes social and environmental factors in its measurement of a nation's well-being, for example, it was clear that climate change and the vulnerability of a broken food system in Hawai'i and Aotearoa New Zealand were the subtext for much of the analysis discussed here. The broad-based appeal of sustainability for most of the interviewees can be traced back to the notion of "doing something positive that localizes the food system and helps minimize carbon emissions" (Lux 2020). Daniela Spoto wrote her graduate thesis on the relationship between climate change, public health, and the food system in 2008, and she explained their mutual impacts were not as evident then as they are now (Spoto 2019). Meleana Judd's family runs a solar business, so she learned from a young age that agriculture contributes to climate change as much as energy consumption does (Judd 2019). Redfeather shared this understanding of conventional agriculture's impact on climate change: "the new awareness about how healthy soils can sequester carbon and be helpful as a soil carbon sponge to help with climate change" (Redfeather 2019). Frieda Lotz-Keegan echoed this sentiment when she said that climate change resilience and carbon sequestration are her passion, because climate resilience and adaptation are necessary to successfully farming any marginal land (Lotz-Keegan 2020). Because she worked in waste reduction, Jacqui Forbes was acutely aware of developed countries' overconsumption habits and decried the economic system that supports this kind of behavior. She said:

> You know, the linear system of take, make, throw away this thing, could only have been created and supported and accepted if it came under a paradigm that was actually not considering water and not considering soil and not considering people. Once we have the right values in place, then I think we can all move optimistically to create a healthier world, planet, peoples. No one can take that power away from us. And you look at where it's got the ecological crisis pushing fading planetary boundaries, hotter, drier climate, you know, dangerous climate change. (Forbes 2020)

Again, this narrative reflects many of the respondents' clear understanding of the larger implications of doing nothing to address food system inequities and their associated environmental problems. Many women expressly mentioned climate change, and for those who didn't, the topic was nonetheless present in their narratives. Jessica Barnes, from one of the Wellington community gardens, reflected on looking at "local solutions for local problems are just gonna get bigger as climate change becomes more of a problem, and this will make all the difference" (Barnes 2020). Even for respondents working in public and community health, climate change was still a key driver to action. Dr. Harwood explained that women notice climate change more because all the evidence suggests that it's going to have the biggest impact on poor people and families with children (Harwood 2020). Barnes and Harwood both reflected on working with mostly Pasifika and Māori women who come to garden throughout the week or come to the marae clinic. Both women saw their stories as bridges to creating connections, maintaining relationships, and addressing climate change by restoring people and places. That cultivation of a sense of place drives community, and therefore climate, resilience. Even the US government's Climate Resilience Toolkit relies on community to plan resilience strategies (2022). The climate crisis is a moment of reckoning for island ecosystems. If we are the "canaries in the coalmine," as it were, then we need to address environmental, public health, and social justice issues by re-valuing Indigenous knowledge systems so that our food systems may represent and serve us all in order to mitigate climate change.

Conclusion

Throughout the narratives, developing policy priorities through community engagement emerged as a critical component of food system work. Community is created through mutual respect and communication, as well as a recognition of the knowledge and skill set each member brings to the collective. Women working together to explore their options for changing the food system exemplify collaborative leadership strategies to formulate AFNs that provide access to good food for everyone. Many of the respondents sought validation in their respective Indigenous cosmologies, not only to honor women's contributions, but also for the strength to redefine success in terms more suited to their communities. Gifts of abundance, not only of food but of knowledge and connections, enables people to establish and maintain resilient food systems in the face of natural, or human-made disasters, like pandemics or climate change. None of this work is easy, and it requires a shift in mindset from short-term political gains or profit motives to long-term visions on the importance of sustainable food systems for healing, both of the land and our bodies.

Conclusions, More Questions, and a Toolkit for Food System Change

Food sovereignty is a feminist issue.
—Elizabeth Mpfou (2020)

It is difficult to write a conclusion about the ongoing transformation of the food system around Oceania, as it is only just beginning. It is not my intention, nor my place, to provide prescriptive solutions, but to weave narratives together to create a coherent vision for food system change. The projects and organizations highlighted in this book are run entirely by women and aimed at creating a healthy, fair, and just food system for all. This is clearly a lofty goal, but if we believe it is too remote, there is a danger we will simply throw up our hands and say that the problems with our food systems are insurmountable. Glib social media comments often admonish people to "do better," but the answer to the question "how?" remains elusive. Change can take the form of large-scale revolution, and it can occur in small, incremental paces. I argue that the stories shared by the women in this project demonstrate that we need both.

The primary solution to combating industrial agriculture and creating a healthy and resilient alternative food system is to focus on soil regeneration. This involves ecological processes that combine Indigenous and agroecological practices centered on nourishing soil and bodies and decolonizing our diets to sustain ourselves and our communities. Food sovereignty is an attainable goal, especially when women are leading the charge. Indigenous "cultures have survived in large part due to the strength of Indigenous women, and it is women who continue to lead today, despite not receiving credit or support" (Gearon 2021). This project attempts to amplify the narrative that women are leading a food system revolution throughout Hawai'i and Aotearoa New Zealand. Even if women in colonized spaces aren't necessarily calling their work feminist, it is apparent that fighting uphill battles on behalf of their families and communities is precisely the kind of grassroots activism that Indigenous feminism calls for.

Intersectional FPE focuses that activism on environmental causes. Those causes are linked to public health, sustainable agriculture, economic development, and thriving communities. They cannot be separated, nor should they be. Cutting-Jones (2020) calls for problematizing colonialism beyond land tenure and economic development by considering gender, indigeneity, race, ethnicity, socioeconomic status, "localness," and foodways. Adding these layers to the analysis provides a fuller and more complex picture of the relationship between neocolonialism and the food system. Cutting-Jones shows that in other Pacific spaces, like the Cook Islands' Rarotonga, women were "resolute leaders who promoted the 'growing of domestic crops'" (2020, 65) for local consumption as opposed to cash crops for export to Aotearoa New Zealand. Cash crops were considered critical to the success of colonial economic development, just as sugarcane and pineapple were in Hawai'i, while families' needs for culturally appropriate food were completely ignored.

It is time for communities to demand action from elected leaders and policymakers. The women interviewed for this project have been doing this exact work. Kelsey Amos, director of the Food + Policy Project, trains college students to become food system activists and leaders. They use the #fixourfoodsystem hashtag to flag and track bills relating to food system issues each legislative session in Hawai'i; this encourages people to submit testimony and learn about the legislative and appropriations processes concerning bills that range from implementing taxes on sugar sweetened beverages to reducing taxes on locally grown *kalo* producers. Amos's leadership is emblematic of the work other women are doing in and around the food system to unsettle colonized spaces, push people's thinking, foster innovation and transformation, and engender empathy and support for the creation of AFNs.

Qualitative interviews necessarily indicate a "point in time" or "snapshot" approach to research. People move on, things change, roles evolve. However, it is a testament to the importance of the work that, a little more than five years after the initial interviews, most of the respondents are still working toward food system transformation in Hawai'i and Aoetaroa New Zealand, respectively. These collective processes inspire others to continue to collaborate to foster change. Many of these women either know of each other, or know each other, but don't always work together. Their voices are not necessarily marginalized, though sometimes they can be. They can also be disconnected, by time or by circumstances. Mona Eltahawy called for those of us who are privileged "to fight ten times harder for those that don't [or can't], to make this platform bigger for the others"

(2016). This project is my effort to do just that. Restoring ancestral abundance of food ways for Kanaka Maoli, Māori, and other marginalized communities is the equivalent of a rising tide that lifts all boats. All communities are better off when Indigenous peoples thrive, especially when living on (and within) island ecosystems threatened by climate change and trying to emerge from centuries of colonial oppression. Restoring the value of Indigenous and traditional ecological knowledges will help restore community and social well-being. Women are leading these efforts, seeking to empower each other and their communities to determine (and share) best practices, achieve food sovereignty, and reshape our current industrial agro-food system geared toward more sustainable community food systems.

As this book has highlighted, Hawai'i and Aotearoa New Zealand are two different island ecosystems in Oceania, both with colonized pasts and a history of land dispossession of Indigenous peoples leading to unsustainable agricultural practices, unchecked development, and corporate power grabs of land and political power. While the American and British colonizers may be different, their strategies were similar with regard to the food system. By taking away access to land, and removing cultural and agricultural practices associated with food, among many other violent strategies of the colonizing process, they reshaped these island nations for their own imperialist purposes.

The responses in each location have been different. Hawai'i has relied on non-profit organizations to address food system injustices and inequities. This work is not necessarily rooted in Kanaka Maoli culture or traditions, although it does often acknowledge and respect it. It primarily aims to reach children through formal institutions like the Department of Education and to reach marginalized communities through health clinics, school lunch programs, educational organizations, and other networks of agricultural communities of practice. The Hawai'i State Legislature, and the various city and county councils on each island, have not been very effective in addressing food system transformation. Thus far, they have opted for very small, incremental changes and provided little support for small farmers or other innovative food system practices like food hubs.

In Aotearoa New Zealand, the politico-legal structure of the ongoing treaty settlements has been effective in enabling food system transformation, though it is not as widespread as it could be. Because each iwi settlement occurs at different times and at different paces depending on the issues at hand, there is no broad overarching policy regarding support for sustainable agriculture. Some Māori iwi have been able to translate their settlements into access to their ancestral lands and fisheries, and have been using them to regenerate ancestral Indigenous abundance for the benefit of their people. This is not the case everywhere, but it does provide a template for Land Back possibilities elsewhere in Oceania, where many other Native peoples continue to resist colonization. This kind of structural change will eventually also lead to social change. It is more of a top-down approach than the grassroots and nonprofit organizing in Hawai'i, but both have potential for success. Ideally, a combination of the two would be the most effective way to achieve food system transformation.

Strategies and Questions for Food System Transformation

Common practices emerged among interviewee narratives and, indeed, the most successful people, projects, and organizations had done the following:

1. Held listening tours of community experts and other stakeholders to determine community needs and existing assets.
2. Embraced authentic, community-specific capacity building.
3. Structured food system resilience projects to be inclusive of local community inputs.
4. Recognized the value of Indigenous agricultural systems.
5. Employed as many best practices from a combination of traditional ecological knowledge and sustainable agriculture.
6. Hawai'i—worked through nonprofits organizations to pull the state along toward food system change.
7. Aotearoa New Zealand—used the existing politico-legal framework of treaty settlements to provide Māori iwi with more space to develop projects for Māori folks to thrive.
8. Creating and maintaining connections among various food system actors are an important part of keeping up momentum for food system transformation.

Common among the many challenges in both Hawai'i and Aotearoa New Zealand were the following:

1. Land-use policy, based on western conceptions of private property in a consumerist and accumulative capitalist system, is a barrier to ahupua'a style land management or Māori-led "moving garden" practices.

2. Hawai'i's lack of recognition of embedded colonization processes makes it difficult to critique the food system from a decolonizing perspective.
3. Wholesale change in the definition of success as it is currently understood in a global capitalist system is necessary. Instead, we should focus on abundance of knowledge, of ancestral wisdom, and of Indigenous values to foster food sovereignty. These are the necessary tools to transform the food system.
4. Talking about decolonization makes some people uncomfortable. It may be easier to talk about food because it's something that everyone has in common, and it is possible not everyone is ready to recognize their role in our respective settler colonial settings. Reframing that narrative around food might be an entryway to that larger discussion.

Even after completing two years of interviews with community experts and food system practitioners, several hurdles to reshaping the food system through an intersectional analysis remain. If we are to rest on the assumption that in order to transform the food system, we must decentralize and re-regionalize our food system, we must acknowledge several barriers. For example, additional agricultural labor is necessary for smaller-scale diversified farming. Reconceptualizing farming as a high-value occupation rather than low-skill, backbreaking labor (while acknowledging that it is, in fact, really hard work) is essential to successful food system transformation. Bringing an intersectional FPE framework to the gendered, raced, classed, aged view of agricultural labor will ensure that society does not reproduce the power and privilege of labor divisions that view manual labor as less valuable than that of the professional classes. Furthermore, higher value labor means that good-tasting, high-quality food costs more. Are people willing to pay more? Does this automatically mean that poor people are not able to afford it? Are we reproducing the currently existing dual class system whereby only some people have access to healthy foods? Could we institutionalize, or even scale up programs like Alicia Higa's Keiki Fresh Fruit and Vegetable Prescription Program at the Wai'anae Coast Comprehensive Health Center, to serve larger segments of the population? Reshaping the food system means reshaping the economy altogether to value important things like good food rather than the overconsumption of environmentally destructive, often government-subsidized foods and goods. The capitalist system is based on the notion of more/bigger: more production, more consumption, more money, more environmental degradation, bigger fruit, bigger vegetables, bigger cows, chickens, and pigs, and bigger farms. All of these stem from the capitalist obsession with economies of scale. Reshaping the food system means basing our economy on the notion of less: smaller farms, less waste, potentially lower yields, but with less negative environmental impacts that would lead to better biodiversity and higher-quality seasonal farm products within smaller regions, reaching more diverse groups of people.

The communities of practice evidenced by the participants in this book have shown that being successful in this work requires the ability to plan, adaptability to changing conditions and/or policies, and openness to working with food system actors in a variety of capacities. Women's leadership in this political resistance to the colonial context is heightened when we hear their stories. The narratives of their lived experiences illustrate the diversity of perspectives and ways in which we can conceptualize food system transformation. This enhances the value of their experiences and shows us how these connections push the boundaries of the possibilities of collaboration. It is important to carefully consider the many possible "what if" scenarios of this work, but here I encourage us to stretch our imaginations as we envision change. What do we want our sustainable community food systems to look like? How can we build food systems so that they serve everyone equitably? What steps can we take to foster this revolution, in this particular political moment? The common denominators here are women, nourishment, resistance, and of course, decolonized food systems. How do we get good food to food insecure places? How do we nourish schoolchildren with culturally appropriate, local, and healthy foods? What do those models look like, and can they be replicated elsewhere? On all the Hawaiian Islands? In Aotearoa New Zealand? Throughout Oceania? So far, the policies in place—as they relate to land use, water rights, Indigenous access to Native lands, and the insistence on cutting costs and supporting economies of scale by relying on the industrial agro-food system—simply have not worked. The result is that a food and agriculture system that worked just fine prior to colonizing European contact is now broken. The current system continues to generate unhealthy people and unhealthy land/soil.

Combining environmental and public health concerns, as well as access to good-tasting and culturally appropriate food, serves justice by reshaping the food system to ensure that everyone has the same opportunities to access what the Slow Food movement originally called "good, clean, and fair food." We are in the middle of a climate crisis and recently lived through a global pandemic—can we see these moments as opportunities to foster change? Can we use what we have learned from and about women's collaborative efforts in Hawai'i and Aotearoa New Zealand to reshape food systems elsewhere? How can Indigenous agricultural and ecological knowledge help us remake our island ecosystems so that they can sustainably feed us? Which other communities in Oceania might have lessons for all of us, in terms of both valuing traditional ecological knowledge and supporting political resistance to colonizing practices? Oceania, with its ancient and innovative migration practices, finite island resources, and connections throughout the commons of the Pacific Ocean, can show the rest of the world that if we can figure out how to fix our broken food systems, other places can too.

GLOSSARY

ahupuaʻa (Hawaiian) – basic unit of land organization in Hawaiian society, varying in size, and forming a connection between mountains and ocean. Contains a variety of resources and were traditionally marked by natural features like streams.

ʻai (Hawaiian) – to eat, enjoy

ʻāina (Hawaiian) – that which feeds; also, sometimes meaning land.

alternative food networks (AFN) – networks of food production defined by short supply chains, local food production, embedded in community, and driven by sustainability; an alternative to conventional, large-scale, highly mechanized, and industrialized agriculture.

ancestral abundance – fostering connection to land and revitalizing traditional Polynesian food practices to enhance community and individual well-being.

Aotearoa New Zealand – referring to the country of New Zealand; using both the Māori term and the English term together highlights the ongoing settler colonial history of the country.

assets-based model – emphasizes strengths and positive attributes of individuals, groups, communities, or systems, rather than focusing on weaknesses and/or deficits.

ahikāroa (Māori) – long-burning fires; represents a concept of continuous occupation of land; signifies a group's traditional connection to land through ancestors who have occupied it for generations.

colonialism – a practice of domination; control of another country or territory, occupying it, subjugating its peoples, and exploiting its resources.

community supported agriculture (CSA) – a partnership between consumers and farmers, where members receive regular deliveries of food, in exchange for an upfront payment, sharing the risks and benefits of local food production.

counterdiscourses – practice of presenting alternative viewpoints or narratives to challenge dominant ideologies or power structures in a society.

counterpublics – members of subordinated social groups invent and circulate counterdiscourses to formulate oppositional interpretations of their identities, interests, and needs.

decolonization – the ongoing process of undoing colonialism, whereby colonies gain independence from colonial powers and transition to self-governance and sovereignty.

deficit-based model – perspective that focuses on the shortcomings or weaknesses of individuals, groups, communities, or systems, attributing failures or limitations to their internal deficiencies rather than external factors or systemic issues.

electronic benefits transfer (EBT) – electronic system used in the United States that allows recipients of government assistance to pay directly for purchases; tends to be used with SNAP (see below) or WIC – Women, Infants, and Children programs to purchase approved food items.

essentialism – the belief that there is a fundamental, inherent "essence" or nature to things or people, often tied to biology or shared psychological traits; criticized for reinforcing stereotypes and excluding diverse experiences.

fair trade – movement and certification system that aims to ensure fair prices, good working conditions, and environmental protection for producers in developing countries.

farm-to-school – initiatives connect local farms with schools to bring fresh, healthy food into school cafeterias and provide students with educational opportunities about agriculture, nutrition, and healthy eating.

feminist food justice – emphasizes feminist leadership in the struggle against the colonial and corporate capture of food systems that extract profits from privatizing the commons, violating human rights, and destroying the environment; fight against patriarchal and neoliberal policies and institutions that hinder women's access to safe, nutritious, and affordable food.

feminist political ecology (FPE) – gendered critical analysis of economic and ecological systems; interrogates structural forms of power that define inequality and differentiated access and control of resources through multiple forms of social difference such as gender, race, class, ethnicity, age, ability, sexuality, and nation.

food desert – a geographically defined area, typically in a low-income, marginalized neighborhood, where residents have limited access to affordable and nutritious food options, particularly fresh fruits and vegetables due either to a lack of transportation or a lack of supermarkets/grocery stores within a convenient distance.

food insecurity – limited or uncertain access to safe, nutritious food for normal growth and development and an active and healthy lifestyle.

food security – consistent access by all people, at all times, to enough safe and nutritious food for a healthy, active life; having physical and economic access to sufficient food that meets people's dietary needs.

food sovereignty – the right of peoples to have healthy and culturally appropriate food, produced through ecologically sound and sustainable methods, and the right to define their own food and agriculture systems.

food system – all the processes and infrastructure involved in feeding a population, from production to consumption; an interconnected web of activities that links food production, processing, distribution, and consumption with human health and the environment.

gender-fluid – denoting or relating to a person who does not identify as having a single unchanging gender; non-fixed gender identity that shifts over time or depending on the situation.

gender non-conforming – denoting or relating to a person whose behavior or appearance does not conform to current prevailing cultural and social expectations about what is appropriate for their gender.

gifting economy – a system of exchange where goods and services are given freely without an explicit expectation of future rewards or remuneration; prioritizes social connections and the act of giving.

globalization – increasing interconnectedness and interdependence of countries' economies, cultures, and populations through the flow of goods, services, technology, and people across borders.

hapū (Māori) – subtribe or clan of an *iwi* (tribe); a grouping of *whānau* (family grouping) who share a common ancestry and often a territory.

Hua Parakore (Māori) – a Māori system and framework for growing *kai* (food) developed by Te Waka Kai Ora (National Māori Organics Authority).

industrial agro-food system – large scale, industrial farming system of crops and animals that emphasizes maximizing output and efficiency through modern technology, mechanization, and chemical inputs; characterized by practices like monoculture farming, heavy chemical use, and reliance on large-scale infrastructure.

intersectionality – theoretical framework that explains how different categories of identity, such as race, gender, class, and sexual orientation, intersect to create unique experiences of discrimination and/or privilege; highlights that individuals are not the sum of their individual identities but that these identities interact and reinforce each other, leading to complex and multifaceted experiences of oppression or advantage.

intersectional praxis – practical application of intersectionality theory into action; involves strategizing and mobilizing intersectionality to develop strategies for social change through collective action that address complex inequalities.

island ecosystem – unique environment, often found on tropical islands, characterized by high biodiversity, endemic species, and distinct evolutionary processes shaped by isolation; may contain many unique plant and animal species.

iwi (Māori) – the largest social unit in Māori society, a tribe that encompasses multiple hapū and whānau. Iwi are often named after a common ancestor or a significant historical event.

kai (Māori) – food or meal; can also be used as a verb meaning to eat or consume.

kaitiakitanga (Māori) – guardianship, care, and protection of the environment, including the land, sea, and sky; responsible stewardship of natural resources, ensuring preservation and sustainability for future generations.

kalo (Hawaiian) – taro; a staple food and plant of great significance in Hawaiian culture; a symbol, a part of the mythology and social structure; kalo is considered the elder brother of mankind, treated with respect and care, reflecting its importance as a food source and symbol of family.

Kanaka Maoli (Hawaiian) – Native Hawaiian (see below); the true people of Hawaiʻi.

Kanaka ʻŌiwi (Hawaiian) – people of the ancestral bone; term used by many Native Hawaiians to self-identify as the original, Indigenous peoples of Hawaiʻi.

kaona (Hawaiian) – hidden meaning or concealed reference; often used in Hawaiian poetry and speech to convey deeper layers of meaning beyond the literal words.

kapu (Hawaiian) – forbidden, sacred, or taboo; a complex system of rules and regulations that governed nearly every aspect of life in Hawaiian society; rules were enforced by chiefs and priests and believed to maintain social order, religious purity, and a balance with the natural world.

kaumātua (Māori) – a senior member of a tribe or community, typically an elder; a term of respect, recognizing the wisdom and experience of older individuals within Māori society.

kaupapa (Māori) – a philosophy or set of principles; plan of action.

keiki (Hawaiian) – baby, child, little one.

kuleana (Hawaiian) – responsibility and privilege; a reciprocal relationship where individuals have a duty to care for and protect the land and community, while also benefiting from reciprocal care and protection offered by the community; a concept that emphasizes shared ownership and interconnectedness; also, a small parcel of land.

kūmara (Māori) – sweet potato; staple food in Māori society.

kupuna (Hawaiian) – elder, grandparent, or ancestor; kūpuna (plural).

Land Back movement – decentralized effort, primarily led by Indigenous peoples, advocating for the return of ancestral lands and resources to Indigenous sovereignty and self-determination; part of a broader movement for decolonization, aiming to rectify historical injustices and establish more equitable systems of land governance.

Mā'awe Pono (Hawaiian) – Hawaiian research methodology focused on decolonization; action research aimed at benefiting Native Hawaiians; developed by Kū Kahakalau in conjunction with thousands of Native Hawaiian co-researchers.

māhele (Hawaiian) – to divide, to portion, to share; also refers to a specific historical process often called the "Great Māhele" of 1848 which marked the transition from a traditional communal land system in Hawai'i to one where individuals could own land privately.

mālama 'āina (Hawaiian) – to respect and care for the land and to properly manage the resources and gifts it provides.

mana (Māori/Hawaiian) – spiritual life force, prestige, authority, and power both in the physical and spiritual realms.

Mana Wahine Māori (Māori) – power, prestige, and authority held by Māori women; framework for understanding and affirming the *mana* of Māori women, both individually and collectively; theory and movement that emphasizes the importance of reclaiming and celebrating the *mana* of Māori women and used to decolonize gender and social structures in Aotearoa.

mana'o (Hawaiian) – thought, idea, belief, opinion, knowledge; a practice of deeply considering and listening to different perspectives when making decisions.

Māori (Māori) – member of the Indigenous peoples of Aotearoa New Zealand; term is not always preferred since it was introduced by colonizers.

marae (Māori) – sacred communal space, often at the heart of a Māori community; serves as a place for religious ceremonies, social gatherings, and formal events; generally associated with a particular iwi, hapū, or whānau.

marae ātea (Māori) – the open space or courtyard in front of the wharenui (meeting house) on a marae; a place where tikanga Māori (customs and protocols) are accorded their ultimate expression.

Native – individuals or groups Indigenous to a particular place or region, meaning they were originally from there and have a strong connection to the land and its culture.

Native Hawaiian – Indigenous people of the Hawaiian Islands, specifically those who are descendants of the aboriginal people who occupied and exercised sovereignty in the area before 1778; term is not always preferred since it was introduced by colonizers.

neocolonialism – control by a state over another nominally independent state, usually a former colony, through indirect means; propagation of socioeconomic and political activity by former colonial rulers aimed at reinforcing capitalism, neoliberal globalization, and cultural subjugation.

neoliberalism – political and economic philosophy that emphasizes free trade, deregulation, globalization, and a reduction in government spending with a focus on economic growth and prosperity.

'ohana (Hawaiian) – family; strong extended network of family, friends, and community, where everyone is valued.

'Ōlelo Hawai'i (Hawaiian) – Hawaiian language; Indigenous language spoken in Hawai'i.

'ōlelo no'eau (Hawaiian) – proverb, poetical or wise saying.

oli (Hawaiian) – chant; a traditional form of expression that was and is still used today in all aspects of life such as acknowledging one's genealogy, honoring a person or place, storytelling, or a protocol before or after certain activities.

organic agriculture – farming system that aims for sustainability and ecological balance by minimizing or eliminating synthetic chemical like pesticides, fertilizers, and genetically modified organisms with a focus on enhancing soil health, biodiversity, and using natural pest control.

Pākehā (Māori) – a person who is not of Māori descent, especially those whose ancestors came from Europe; a white person.

Polynesia – from the Greek for "many islands" a collection of over 1,000 islands in the Pacific Ocean; set within a geographic triangle formed by Aotearoa New Zealand in the southwest, Rapa Nui (Easter Island) in the southeast, and the Hawaiian archipelago in the north.

rangatiratanga (Māori) – chieftainship, right to exercise authority; later also Indigenous self-determination; the right of Māori people to rule themselves.

regenerative agriculture – a farming approach that focuses on improving soil health and ecological systems to increase productivity, biodiversity, and resilience to climate change; reduces water use and other inputs; conservation and rehabilitation approach to food and farming systems.

settler colonialism – ongoing system of power that perpetuates the genocide and repression of Indigenous peoples and cultures.

strategic essentialism – a political tactic where marginalized groups highlight shared identities to mobilize for political action, even if those identities are seen as constructed or simplified; temporary use of essentialism to affirm and consolidate political identities; flexible and adaptable tool that allows groups to navigate complex power dynamics by strategically using and sometimes subverting the concept of essential identity.

subaltern – a person holding inferior rank or a subordinate position; groups in society who are subject to the hegemony of the ruling classes and have been marginalized or oppressed.

Supplemental Nutrition Assistance Program (SNAP) – federal program funded through the US Department of Agriculture; provides crucial food and nutritional support to qualifying low-income and needy households, and those making the transition from welfare to self-sufficiency.

sustainable agriculture – a farming approach that focuses on long-term conservation of natural resources and environmentally-friendly practices while meeting the present and future food needs of society, without compromising the ability of future generations to do the same.

talk story (Hawaiʻi Creole English/Pidgin) – talking with old friends, passing time by chit-chatting, or rekindling old times; to chat informally, or "shoot the breeze."

tangata whenua (Māori) – people of the land; refers to the Indigenous Māori people and their connection to the land, either to a specific region or to Aotearoa New Zealand as a whole.

te ao Māori (Māori) – Maori worldview.

Te Reo Māori (Māori) – the native language of Aotearoa New Zealand; the language of the Indigenous Māori people.

terroir (French) – earth or soil; a cultivated ecosystem in which grapevines interact with factors from the natural environment, principally soil and climate; generally used when referring to wine but can be applied to other agricultural products growing in the soil.

Te Tiriti O Waitangi/Treaty of Waitangi (Māori/English) – agreement made in 1840 between representatives of the British Crown and more than 500 *rangatira* Māori (Māori chiefs) and resulted in declaration of British sovereignty over Aotearoa New Zealand; the English treaty and the Te Reo tiriti held different meanings and Māori and Pākehā had different expectations of the treaty's terms.

tikanga (Māori) – traditional customary practices, behaviors and principles that guide Māori social interactions and cultural understanding; encompasses a framework for appropriate conduct, promoting respect, and demonstrating cultural sensitivity.

tūrangawaewae (Māori) – a place to stand and belong; a feeling of home, a connection to a particular place.

ʻ*ulu* (Hawaiian) – scientific name: *Artocarpus altilis*; breadfruit; a starchy tree fruit; a staple food throughout Oceania; considered a symbol of resilience and sustainability.

ʻ*uala* (Hawaiian) – scientific name: *Ipomoea batatas*; sweet potato; popular and versatile ingredient in Hawaiian cuisine.

wairua (Māori) – spirit, soul, or spiritual dimension of a person, entity, or place; in Māori worldview, connection to the spiritual realm and the essence of being.

whakapapa (Māori) – genealogy, lineage, descent; represents the tracing of one's ancestry and connections to the past, present, and future; encompasses a broad understanding of connections between people, land, and the universe.

whānau (Māori) – extended family, family group; includes immediate family, foster children, and even those who have passed on; primary economic and social unit of traditional Māori society.

whenua (Māori) – land, country, territory; placenta, reflecting deep connection between land and people, similar to the umbilical cord linking a child to its mother.

women – individuals who identify as female.

LIST OF INTERVIEWEES

Allen, Trish. (2020). Co-founder, Rainbow Valley Farm. Matakana, Aotearoa New Zealand.

Albrecht, Kristin. (2019). Executive Director, The Food Basket. Hilo, Hawai'i Island.

Barnes, Jessica. (2020). Garden manager, For The Better Good Community and Market Garden. Wellington, Aotearoa New Zealand.

Baxter, Kay. (2020). Co-Founder, Kōanga Seed Saving Institute. Wairoa, Aotearoa New Zealand.

Bowen, Hilary. (2020). Co-owner, The Front Room Cafe. Waikanae Beach, Aotearoa New Zealand.

Brinker, Amy. (2019). Director of Sustainability, Kamehameha Schools. Honolulu, O'ahu.

Burchard, Sarah. (2019). Freelance food writer and journalist. Honolulu, O'ahu.

Carlson, Laurie. (2019). Co-founder, Kokua Market and co-founder of Slow Food Hawai'i. Honolulu, O'ahu.

Cherrington, Kate. (2020). Chair of Te Pūtea Whakatupu Trust (now known as Tapuwae Roa). Wellington, Aotearoa New Zealand.

Clifford, Angela. (2020). Chief Executive Officer, Eat New Zealand. Waipara Valley, North Canterbury, Aotearoa New Zealand.

Cole, Betsy. (2019). Deputy Director, The Kohala Center. Waimea, Hawai'i Island.

Esquivel, Monica. (2019). Assistant Professor of Dietetics, University of Hawai'i at Mānoa, Board Member, Good Food Alliance. Honolulu, O'ahu.

Forbes, Jacqui. (2020). Director, Xtreme Zero Waste. Raglan/Whāingaroa, Aotearoa New Zealand.

Francis, Kelly. (2020). Founder, Whenua Warrior. Auckland, Aotearoa New Zealand.

Geller, Nanette. (2019). Supplemental Assistance to Needy Families/Electronic Benefits Transfer Coordinator, Hawaiʻi Farm Bureau Farmers' Markets. Honolulu, Oʻahu.

Harwood, Matire. (2020). University of Auckland Medical and Health Sciences Faculty and general practitioner at Papakura Marae Health Clinic. Papakura, Auckland, Aotearoa New Zealand.

Higa, Alicia. (2019). Director of Health Promotion, Waiʻanae Coast Comprehensive Health Center. Waiʻanae, Oʻahu.

Hitchens, Moulika. (2019). Staff, Health Promotion, Waiʻanae Coast Comprehensive Health Center. Waiʻanae, Oʻahu.

Huff, Lehn. (2019). Member, Maui School Garden Network. Maui.

Judd, Meleana. (2019). Owner, Waihuena Farm, North Shore, Oʻahu.

Keegan, Ness. (2020). Co-Owner, PermaDynamics Farm. Te Tai Tokerau, Aotearoa New Zealand.

King, Emily. (2020). Founder, Spira NZ and author of *Re-Food*. Aotearoa, New Zealand.

Koethe, Frankie. (2019). Natural Resources Specialist, Oʻahu Resources Defense Council. Kunia, Oʻahu.

Ladrig, Rachel. (2019). Farm Coach, GoFarm Hawaiʻi, formerly at Kahumana Farms and Farmers' Union United. Windward Oʻahu.

Lotz-Keegan, Frieda. (2020). Co-Owner, PermaDynamics Farm. Te Tai Tokerau, Aotearoa New Zealand.

Lukens, Ashley. (2019). Hawaiʻi Center for Food Safety, co-founder Hawaiʻi Food Policy Council. Honolulu, Oʻahu.

Lux, Jenny. (2020). Owner, Lux Organics Farm. Rotorua, Aotearoa New Zealand.

Maunakea, Summer. (2019). Assistant Professor of Curriculum Studies, College of Education, University of Hawai'i at Mānoa. Honolulu, O'ahu.

Morgan-Bernal, Lydi. (2020). Hawai'i Farm-to-School Coordinator. Honolulu, O'ahu.

Mules, Rangimārie. (2020). Co-director, Oi Collective, Ltd. Aotearoa New Zealand

Oddom, Ka'iulani. (2019). Roots Program Director, Kōkua Kalihi Valley Community Health Center. Kalihi, O'ahu.

Oshiro, Joleen. (2019). Food Writer. *Honolulu Star Advertiser*. Kapolei, O'ahu.

Redfeather, Nancy. (2019). Kū 'Āina Pā Education Program Director, Kohala Center. Waimea, Hawai'i Island.

Rohr, Jessica. (2019). Founder and Owner, Forage Hawai'i. Honolulu, O'ahu.

Ropati, Hineamaru. (2020). Hua Parakore teacher, Papatūānuku Kōkiri Marae. South Auckland, Aotearoa New Zealand.

Samson, Ku'ulei. Director of Educational Programs, Hoa 'Āina O Mākaha. Mākaha, O'ahu.

Sana, Kaui. (2019). Farm manager, MA'O Farms. Wai'anae, O'ahu.

Shapiro, Dana. (2019). Executive Director, 'Ulu Cooperative. Kailua-Kona, Hawai'i Island.

Skelton, Pounamu (2020). Hua Parakore teacher. Te Ati Awa, Taranaki, Aotearoa New Zealand.

Smith, Tammy. (2019). Dietary Manager, King Lunalilo Trust and Home. Honolulu, O'ahu.

Smuts-Kennedy, Sarah. (2020). Founder, For the Love of Bees and artist. Auckland, Aotearoa New Zealand.

Spoto, Daniela. (2019). Director of Food Equity. Hawai'i Appleseed Center for Law and Economic Justice. Honolulu, O'ahu.

Sullivan, Claire. (2019). Chief Executive Officer, Farm Link Hawai'i. Honolulu, O'ahu.

Tait-Jameson, Cathy (2020). Co-founder, BioFarm Dairy. Palmerston North. Aotearoa New Zealand.

Tamai, Tina. (2019). Executive Director, Hawai'i Good Food Alliance. Honolulu, O'ahu.

Wamsley, Kate. (2020). Director of Compost Program, Kaicycle. Wellington, Aotearoa New Zealand.

Watts, Ashley. (2019). Owner, Local 'Ia Fishery. Honolulu, O'ahu.

Williams, Harmonee. (2019). Co-founder and Executive Director of Sust'āinable Molokai. Kaunakakai, Moloka'i.

Zwartz, Hannah. (2020). Master gardener and educator, Urban Kai. Lower Hutt, Aotearoa New Zealand.

WORKS CITED

Adams, C. J. 1990. *The Sexual Politics of Meat: A Feminist-Vegetarian Critical Theory*. Continuum.

Adams, D.C. & Salois, M.J. 2010. "Local Versus Organic: A Turn in Consumer Preferences and Willingness-to-pay." *Renewable Agriculture and Food Systems*, 25, 331-341. https://doi.org/10.1017/S1742170510000219.

Agarwal, B. 1994. *A Field of One's Own: Gender and Land Rights in South Asia.* Cambridge University Press.

Agarwal, B. 2014. "Food Sovereignty, Food Security and Democratic Choice: Critical Contradictions, Difficult Conciliations." *Journal of Peasant Studies* 41 (6): 1247–1268. https://doi.org/10.1080/03066150.2013.876996.

Aguayo, B. C. & A. Latta. 2015. "Agro-ecology and Food Sovereignty Movements in Chile: Sociospatial Practices for Alternative Peasant Futures." *Annals of the Association of American Geographers* 105 (2): 397–406. https://doi.org/10.1080/00031870.2015.1045064.

Aikau, H.K. & Gonzalez, V.V. eds. 2019. *Detours: A Decolonial Guide to Hawai'i.* Duke University Press.

'Āina Momona. 2025. "'Ōlelo No'eau About Land." https://www.kaainamomona.org/olelo-noeau-land.

Alanes, M. N. 2022. "Dairy in the Americas: How Colonialism Left its Mark on the Continent." https://sentientmedia.org/dairy-in-the-americas-how-colonialism-left-its-mark-on-the-continent/.

Alcoff, L. 1991. "The Problem of Speaking for Others." *Cultural Critique* 20: 5–32. https://doi.org/10.2307/1354221.

Alfred, T. 2002. "Sovereignty." In *A Companion to American Indian History*, edited by P.J. Deloria & N. Salisbury. Blackwell Publishing.

Alfred, T. & Corntassel, J. 2005. "Being Indigenous: Resurgences against Contemporary Colonialism." *Government and Opposition* 40 (4): 597–614. https://doi.org/10.1111/j.1477-7053.2005.00166.x.

Alkon, A.H. & Norgaard, K.M. 2009. "Breaking the Food Chains: An Investigation of Food Justice Activism." *Sociological Inquiry* 79 (3): 289–305. https://doi.org/10.1111/j.1475-682X.2009.00291.x.

Allen, P. 2004. *Together at the Table: Sustainability and Sustenance in the American Agrifood System.* Pennsylvania University Press.

Allen, P. & Sachs, C.E. 1992. "The Poverty of Sustainability: An Analysis of Current Positions." *Agriculture and Human Values* 9 (4): 29–35. https://doi.org/10.1007/bf02217962.

Allen, P. & Sachs, C.E. 2007. "Women and Food Chains: The Gendered Politics of Food." *International Journal of Sociology of Food and Agriculture* 15 (1): 1–23. https://www.ijsaf.org/index.php/ijsaf/article/view/424.

Alvarez, L. 2022. "Colonization, Food, and the Practice of Eating." *Food Empowerment Project.* https://foodispower.org/our-food-choices/colonization-food-and-the-practice-of-eating/.

American Meat Institute. 2025. "The Power of Meat." https://www.meatinstitute.org/press/sales-record-high-americans-view-meat-part-healthy-balanced-lifestyle-power-meat-analysis.

Anderson, J. 2013. "The Empire Bites Back? Writing Food in Oceania." *Portal Journal of Multidisciplinary Studies* 10 (2): 1–17. https://doi.org/10.5130/portal.v10i2.3067.

Avakian A. & Haber, B. 2006. "Feminist Food Studies: A Brief History." In *From Betty Crocker to Feminist Food Studies: Critical Perspectives on Women and Food,* edited by A. Avakian & B. Haber. University of Massachusetts Press.

Ban Ki-Moon. 2013. *Global Strategy for Women and Children's Health.* Routledge.

Barber, D. 2015. *The Third Plate: Field Notes on the Future of Food.* Penguin.

Barnes, K.L., & Bendixsen, C.G. 2017. "'When this Breaks Down, it's Black Gold': Race and Gender in Agricultural Health and Safety." *Journal of Agromedicine* 22 (1): 56–65. https://doi.org/10.1080/1059924X.2016.1251368.

Barreca, R. 2020. Founder, Farm Link Hawai'i. Personal Communication.

Bartos, A. 2016. "Food Sovereignty and the Possibilities for an Equitable, Just and Sustainable Food System." *In Eating, Drinking: Surviving*, edited by P. Jackson, W. Spiess & F. Sultana. Springer Briefs in Global Understanding. Springer.

Bean, M., & Sharp, J. S. 2011. "Profiling Alternative Food System Supporters: The Personal and Social Basis of Local and Organic Food Support." *Renewable Agriculture and Food Systems*, 26 (3), 243–254. http://www.jstor.org/stable/44490657.

Bergman, M.M. 2020. "'We're at a Crossroads': Who Do the Fish of Hawaii Belong To?" *The Guardian.* https://www.theguardian.com/environment/2020/aug/26/hawaii-fish-waters-native-commercial-fishers.

Belfi, E., & Sandiford, N. 2021. "Decolonization Part 3: Land Back." In *Interdependence: Global Solidarity and Local Actions,* edited by S. Brandauer & E. Hartman. The Community Based Learning Collaborative.

Berry, W. 2009. "The Pleasures of Eating." *Ecoliteracy Magazine.* https://www.ecoliteracy.org/article/wendell-berry-pleasures-eating.

Biodynamic Association. 2024. "Biodynamic Principles and Practices." https://www.biodynamics.com/biodynamic-principles-and-practices.

Blair, C. 2020. "Are You Local? What These Hawaii Scholars Have to Say Might Surprise You." *Civil Beat.* https://www.civilbeat.org/2020/01/are-you-local-what-these-hawaii-scholars-have-to-say-might-surprise-you/.

Blum, S. D. 2011–2012. "Called by the Earth: Women in Sustainable Farming." *Journal of Workplace Rights* 16 (3–4): 315–336. https://doi.org/10.2190/wr.16.3-4.d.

Bosco, F. & Joassart-Marcelli, P. 2018. "Relational Space and Place and Food Environments: Geographic Insights for Critical Sustainability Research." *Journal of Environmental Studies and Sciences* 8 (4): 539–546. https://doi.org/10.1007/s13412-018-0482-9.

Butalia, U. 2000. *The Other Side of Silence: Voices from the Partition of India.* Duke University Press.

Butler, J. 1990. *Gender Trouble: Feminism and the Subversion of Identity.* Routledge.

Byrd, J.A. 2011. *The Transit of Empire: Indigenous Critiques of Colonialism.* University of Minnesota Press.

Cairns, K., Johnston, J. & Baumann, S. 2010. "Caring about Food: Doing Gender in the Foodie Kitchen." *Gender and Society* 24 (5): 591–615. https://doi.org/10.1177/0891243210383419.

Castellano, R.L.S. 2015. "Alternative Food Networks and Food Provisioning as a Gendered Act." *Agriculture and Human Values* 21: 461–474. https://doi.org/10.1007/s10460-014-9562-y.

Castellano, R.L.S. 2016. "Alternative Food Networks and the Labor of Food Provisioning: A Third Shift?" *Rural Sociology* 81 (3): 445–469. https://doi.org/10.1111/ruso.12104.

Centers for Disease Control. 2023. "Tips for Healthy Eating for a Healthy Weight." *Healthy Weight and Growth.* https://www.cdc.gov/healthy-weight-growth/healthy-eating/index.html.

Chiappe, M.B. & Flora, C.B. 1998. "Gendered Elements of the Alternative Agriculture Paradigm." *Rural Sociology* 63 (3): 372–393. https://doi.org/10.1111/j.1549-0831.1998.tb00684.x.

Cho, S., Crenshaw, K.W. & McCall, L. 2013. "Toward a Field of Intersectionality Studies: Theory, Applications, and Praxis." *Signs* 38(4), 785–810. https://doi.org/10.1086/669608.

Coaston, J. 2019. "The Intersectionality Wars." *Vox.com*, May 28. https://www.vox.com//the-highlight/2019/5/20/18542843/intersectionality-conservatism-law-race-gender-discrimination.

Companies Market Cap. 2025. "Revenue for Fonterra." https://companiesmarketcap.com/fonterra/revenue/.

Costa, L.R. & Besio, K. 2011. "Eating Hawai'i: Local Foods and Place-Making in Hawai'i Regional Cuisine." *Social & Cultural Geography* 12 (8): 839–854. https://doi.org/10.1080/14649365.2011.615664.

Coté, C. 2016. "'Indigenizing' Food Sovereignty: Revitalizing Indigenous Food Practices and Ecological Knowledges in Canada and the United States." *Humanities* 5 (3): 12–57. https://doi.org/10.3390/h5030057.

Crenshaw, K. 1991. "Mapping the Margins: Intersectionality, Identity Politics, and Violence Against Women of Color." *Stanford Law Review* 43, 1241–1299. https://doi.org/10.2307/1229039.

Chrisman, S. 2025. "The Food Print of Dairy." https://foodprint.org/reports/the-foodprint-of-dairy/.

Cutting-Jones, H. 2020. "The Conscience of the Community: The Au Vaine of Rarotonga." *Journal of Pacific History* 55 (1): 58–79. https://doi.org/10.108 0/00223344.2019.1636215.

Daigle, M. 2017. "Tracing the Terrain of Indigenous Food Sovereignties." *Journal of Peasant Studies.* http://dx.doi.org/10.1080/03066150.2017.1324423.

Dairy Companies Association of New Zealand. 2020. "About the New Zealand Dairy Industry." https://www.dcanz.com/about-the-nz-dairy-industry/.

Daly, M. 1978. *Gyn/Ecology: The Metaethics of Radical Feminism.* Beacon Press.

Danius , S., Jonsson, S. & Spivak , G.C. 1993. "An Interview with Gayatri Chakravorty Spivak." *Boundary 2*, 20 (2): 24–50. https://doi.org/10.2307/303357.

David Suzuki Foundation. 2023. What Is Land Back? https://davidsuzuki.org/what-you-can-do/what-is-land-back/.

Davis, B., Lipper, L. & Winters, P. 2022. "Do Not Transform Food Systems on the Backs of the Rural Poor." *Food Security* 14: 729–740. https://doi.org/10.1007/s12571-021-01214-3.

Deer, S. 2015. *The Beginning and End of Rape: Confronting Sexual Violence in Native America.* University of Minnesota Press.

DeLind, L.B. 2010. "Are Local Food and the Local Food Movement Taking Us Where We Want To Go? Or Are We Hitching our Wagons to the Wrong Stars?" *Agriculture and Human Values* 28 (2): 273–283. https://doi.org/10.1007/s10460-010-9263-0.

DeLind, L.B. & Ferguson, A. 1999. "Is this a Women's Movement? The Relationship of Gender to Community Supported Agriculture in Michigan." *Human Organization* 58 (2): 190–200. https://doi.org/10.17730/humo.58.2.lpk17625008871x7.

Dempsey, R.C., McAlaney, J. & Bewick, B.M. 2018. "A Critical Appraisal of the Social Norms Approach as an Interventional Strategy for Health-Related Behavior and Attitude Change." *Frontiers in Psychology* 9. https://doi.org/10.3389/fpsyg.2018.02180.

Deutsch, T. 2011. "Memories of Mothers in the Kitchen: Local Foods, History, and Women's Work." *Radical History Review* 110: 167–177. https://doi.org/10.1215/01636545-2010-032.

Duvauchelle, J. 2019. "Seeing Ethical Meat Through an Indigenous Lens: Hunting for a More Sustainable Future." *Alive*, October 30. https://www .alive.com/lifestyle/seeing-ethical-meat-through-an-indigenous-lens.

d'Eaubonne, Françoise. 1974. *Le Féminisme Ou la Mort/Feminism or Death.* P. Horay.

Edwards-Jones, G. 2010. "Does Eating Local Food Reduce the Environmental Impact of Food Production and Enhance Consumer Health?" *Proceedings of the Nutrition Society* 69: 582–591. https://doi.org/10.1017/s0029665110002004.

Eltahawy, M. 2016. "Be the Revolution: Mona Eltahawy interviewed by Chinaka Hodge." https://www.youtube.com/watch?v=cvjSa90bUWw.

Enos, K. 2013. "Working Collectively to Restore Ancestral Abundance." UH Mānoa TEDx Talk. https://www.youtube.com/watch?v=w8iou8Rchqc.

Environmental Protection Agency. 2022. "Sources of Greenhouse Gas Emissions. " https://www.epa.gov/ghgemissions/sources-greenhouse-gas-emissions.

Escurriol, M.V. & Rosa y Rivera-Ferre Binimelis, M.G. 2014. "The Situation of Rural Women in Spain: The Case of Small-scale Artisan Food Producers." *Athenea Digital* 14 (3): 3–22. https://doi.org/10.5565/rev/athenead/v14n3.1186.

Esquibel, C. R. & Calvo, L. 2013. "Decolonize your Diet: A Manifesto." *Nineteen Sixty-Nine: An Ethnic Studies Journal* 2 (1): 1–5. https://escholarship. org/uc/item/7wb1d2t6.

Esquivel, M.K., Higa, A., Hitchens, M., Shelton, C. & Okihiro, M. 2020. "Keiki Produce Prescription (KPRx) Program Feasibility Study to Reduce Food Insecurity and Obesity Risk." *Hawaiʻi Journal of Health & Social Welfare* 79 (5 Suppl 1): 44–49. https://pmc.ncbi.nlm.nih.gov/articles/PMC7260871/.

Evans, R. 2019. "The Negation of Powerlessness: Māori Feminism, a Perspective." In *Mana Wahine Reader: A Collection of Writings 1987–1998*, vol. I, edited by L. Pihama, L. Tuhiwai Smith, N. Simmonds, J. Seed-Pihama & K. Gabel. Te Kotahi Research Institute.

Feldman, S. & Welsh, R. 1995. "Feminist Knowledge Claims, Local Knowledge, and Gender Divisions of Agricultural Labor: Constructing a Successor Science." *Rural Sociology* 60 (1): 23–43. https://doi.org/10.1111/j.1549-0831.1995.tb00561.x.

Fellezs, K. 2019. *Listen but Don't Ask Question: Hawaiian Slack Key Guitar Across the TransPacific.* Duke University Press.

Fielding-Singh, P. 2017. "A Taste of Inequality: Food's Symbolic Value Across the Socioeconomic Spectrum." *Sociological Science* 4: 424–448. https://doi .org/10.15195/v4.a17.

Finney, B. 1996. "Colonizing an Island World." *Transactions of the American Philosophical Society* 86 (5): 71–116. https://doi.org/10.2307/1006622.

Fraser, N. 1990. "Rethinking the Public Sphere: A Contribution to the Critique of Actually Existing Democracy." *Social Text* 25: 56–80. https://doi .org/10.2307/466240.

Gaard, G., ed. 1993. *Ecofeminism: Women, Animals, Nature.* Temple University Press.

Gaard, G. 2013. *International Perspectives in Feminist Ecocriticism.* Routledge.

Gearon, J. 2021. "Indigenous Feminism is our Culture." *Stanford Social Innovation Review*, February 21. https://ssir.org/articles/entry/indigenous_feminism_is_our_culture.

Gillespie, K. 2014. "Feminist Food Politics." In *Macmillan Interdisciplinary Handbook Series* (MHIS) – Gender, 2nd ed: 149-163. Cengage Learning.

Glickman, A. 2019. "Poetry as Protest: Adrienne Rich Fought for All Women." *Jewish Women's Archive.* https://jwa.org/blog/risingvoicespoetry-as-protest-adrienne-rich-fought-for-all-women.

Glover, M., Wong, S.F., Taylor, R.W., Derraik, J.G.B., Faʻalili-Fidow, J., Morton, S.M. & Cutfield, W.S. 2019. "The Complexity of Food Provisioning Decisions by Māori Caregivers to Ensure the Happiness and Health of their Children." *Nutrients* 11: 994. https://doi.org/10.3390/nu11050994.

GoFarm Hawaiʻi. 2025. "Do You Need to Develop Necessary Farming Skills?" https://gofarmhawaii.org/develop-necessary-skills/.

Goodman, D. 2004. "Rural Europe Redux? Reflections on Alternative Agro-food Networks and Paradigm Change." *Sociologia Ruralis* 44 (1): 3–16. https://doi .org/10.1111/j.1467-9523.2004.00258.x.

Goodman, D., & DuPuis, M. 2002. "Knowing Food and Growing Food: Beyond the Production-Consumption Debate in the Sociology of Agriculture." *Sociologia Ruralis* 42 (1): 5–22. https://doi.org/10.1111/1467-9523.00199.

Goodman, D. & Goodman, M. 2009. "Alternative Food Networks." In *International Encyclopedia of Human Geography*, edited by R. Kitchin & N. Thrift. Elsevier.

Goodyear-Ka'ōpua, N., Hussey, N.I., & Wright, E.K., eds. 2014. *A Nation Rising: Hawaiian Movements for Life, Land and Sovereignty*. Duke University Press.

Grandin, T. ed. 2021. *Improving Animal Welfare: A Practical Approach,* 3rd ed. CAB International.

Griffin, S. 1978. *Woman and Nature: The Roaring Inside Her*. Harper & Row.

Grimshaw, P. 1989. *Paths of Duty: American Missionary Wives and Nine-teenth-Century Hawaii*. University of Hawai'i Press.

Gupta, C. 2018. "Dairy's Decline and the Politics of 'Local Milk' in Hawai'i." In *The Foodways of Hawai'i: Past and Present*, edited by H.J. Hobart: 59-90. Routledge.

Guthman, J. 2007. "'Can't Stomach It': How Michael Pollan et al. Made Me Want to Eat Cheetos." *Gastronomica: The Journal of Food and Culture* 3: 75-79. https://doi.org/10.1525/gfc.2007.7.3.75.

Guthman, J. 2008. "Bringing Good Food to Others: Investigating the Subjects of Alternative Food Practice." *Cultural Geographies* 15 (4): 431-447. https://doi.org/10.1177/1474474008094315.

Guthman, J. 2011. "If They Only Knew: The Unbearable Whiteness of Alternative Food." In *Cultivating Food Justice: Race, Class and Sustainability*, edited by A.H. Alkon, & J. Agyeman. Massachusetts Institute of Technology.

Guthman, J., Morris, A., & Allen, P. 2006. "Squaring Farm Security and Food Security in Two Types of Alternative Food Institutions." *Rural Sociology* 71 (4): 662–684. https://doi.org/10.1526/003601106781262034.

Hale, L. Z. & Rude, J. eds. 2017. *Learning from New Zealand's 30 Years of Experience Managing Fisheries Under a Quota Management System*. The Nature Conservancy.

Hancock, F. 2021a. "What Dairy Farming is Doing to NZ's Water." *Radio New Zealand.* https://www.rnz.co.nz/news/whoseatingnewzealand/447861/what-dairy-farming-is-doing-to-nz-s-water.

Hancock, F. 2021b. "Who's Eating New Zealand?" https://www.stuff.co.nz/business/farming/300350351/whos-eating-new-zealand.

Haraway, D. 1998. "Situated Knowledges: The Science Question in Feminism and the Privilege of Partial Perspective." *Feminist Studies* 14 (3): 575–599. https://doi.org/10.2307/3178066.

Harvard School of Public Health. 2017. "Harvard Researchers Continue to Support their Healthy Eating Plate." *Harvard Health Publications.* https://www. health.harvard.edu/staying-healthy/harvard-researchers-launch-healthy-eating-plate.

Hauʻofa, E. 1994. "Our Sea of Islands." *Contemporary Pacific* 6 (1): 148–161. http://www.jstor.org/stable/23701593.

Hawaiʻi Tourism Authority Research and Economic Analysis Division. 2025. "Visitor Industry Continued Improvement in December 2024." *Hawaiʻi Department of Business, Economic Development, and Tourism.* https://www. hawaiitourismauthority.org/research/monthly-visitor-statistics/.

Hawaiigoodfoodalliance.org. 2022. "Hawaiʻi Good Food Alliance: About Us." https://hawaiigoodfoodalliance.org/about/.

Hawaiipublicschools.org. 2022. "State Reports." https://hawaiipublicschools. org/data-reports/state-reports/.

Hawaiʻi Social Epigenomics Early Diabetes Cohort. 2021. "The Study." https:// hiseed.org/research.

Healthy Families NZ. 2023. "Healthy Families NZ "Community Up" Approach to Improving Wellbeing and Equity." Commissioning for *Pae Ora: Healthy Futures Case Study*, edited by Ministry of Health. Wellington: Ministry of Health.

Heaton, T. 2022. "The Deer Population is Devastating Maui: Hunters Want to Help." *Civil Beat.* https://www.civilbeat.org/2022/03/the-deer-population-is-devastating-maui-hunters-want-to-help/.

Hernandez, I. 2022. "What is White Veganism?" https://queerbrownvegan. com/what-is-white/veganism/.

Hill Collins, P. & Bilge, S. 2020. *Intersectionality: Key Concepts* (2nd ed). Polity Press.

Hill Collins, P. 1990. *Black Feminist Thought: Knowledge, Consciousness, and the Politics of Empowerment.* Unwin Hyman.

Hinrichs, C.C. & Kremer, K. 2002. "Social Inclusion in a Midwest Local Food System Project." *Journal of Poverty* 6: 65–90. https://doi.org/10.1300/J134v06n01_04.

Hofman, N.G. 2016. "Bridging Food Scarcity: Croatian Women's Responses to Consumer Capitalism." *Culture, Agriculture, Food and Environment* 38 (1): 48–56. https://doi.org/10.1111/cuag.12065.

Holloway, L., Kneafsey, M., Venn, L., Cox, R., Dowler, E., & Tuomainen, H. 2007. "Possible Food Economies: A Methodological Framework for Exploring Food Production-Consumption Relationships." *Sociologia Ruralis* 47 (1): 1–19. https://doi.org/10.1111/j.1467-9523.2007.00427.x

hooks, b. 1984. *Feminist Theory from Margin to Center.* South End Press.

Hovorka, A.J. 2023. "Exploring Urban Foodscapes via Feminist Political Ecology." In *Routledge Handbook of Urban Food Governance*, edited by Moragues-Faus, A., Clark J.K., Battersby, J. & Davies, A. Routledge.

Huambachano, M.A. 2018. "Enacting Food Sovereignty in Aotearoa New Zealand and Peru: Revitalizing Indigenous Knowledge, Food Practices and Ecological Philosophies." *Journal of Agroecology and Sustainable Food Systems* 42 (9): 1003–1028. https://doi.org/10.1080/21683565.2018.1468380.

Huambachano, M.A. 2019. "Indigenous Food Sovereignty: Reclaiming Food as Sacred Medicine in New Zealand and Peru." *New Zealand Journal of Ecology* 43(3): 3383. https://dx.doi.org/10.20417/nzjecol.43.39.

Hutchings, N.J. 2015. *Te Mahi Māra Hua Parakore: A Māori Food Sovereignty Handbook.* Te Tākupu, Te Wānanga o Raukawa.

Immerwahr, D. 2019. *How to Hide an Empire: A History of the Greater United States.* Farrar, Strauss and Giroux.

Indigenous Women's Network. 2009. In *Encyclopedia of Gender and Society* edited by J. O'Brien: 459-459. https://doi.org/10.4135/9781412964517.n228.

Innes-Gold, A.A., Madin, E., Stokes, K., Ching, C., Kawelo, H., Kotubetey, K., Reppun, F., Rii, Y.M., Winter, K.B., & McManus, L.C. 2024. "Restoration of an Indigenous Aquaculture System can Increase Reef Fish Density and Fisheries Harvest in Hawaiʻi." *Ecosphere.* https://doi.org/10.1002/ecs2.4797.

Irwin, K. 2019. "Towards Theories of Māori Feminisms." In *Mana Wahine Reader: A Collection of Writings 1987–1998*, vol. I, edited by L. Pihama, L. Tuhiwai Smith, N. Simmonds, J. Seed-Pihama & K. Gabel. Te Kotahi Research Institute.

Jacob, M M. 2010. "Claiming Health and Culture as Human Rights: Yakama Feminism in Daily Practice." *International Feminist Journal of Politics* 12 (3–4): 361–380. https://doi.org/10.1080/14616742.2010.513106.

Jarosz, L. 2014. "Comparing Food Security and Food Sovereignty Discourses." *Dialogues in Human Geography* 4(2): 168-181. https://doi.org/10.1177/2043820614537161.

Joassart-Marcelli, P. & Bosco F.J., eds. 2018. *Food and Place: A Critical Exploration*. Rowman & Littlefield.

Johnston, P. & Pihama, L. 2019. "What Counts as Difference and What Differences Count: Gender, Race and the Politics of Difference." In *Mana Wahine Reader: A Collection of Writings 1987–1998*, vol. I, edited by L. Pihama, L. Tuhiwai Smith, N. Simmonds, J. Seed-Pihama & K. Gabel. Te Kotahi Research Institute.

Jones, R., Wham, C. & Burlingame, B. 2019. "New Zealand's Food System is Unsustainable: A Survey of the Divergent Attitudes of Agriculture, Environment, and Health Sector Professionals Towards Eating Guidelines." *Frontiers in Nutrition* 6: 99. https://doi.org/10.3389/fnut.2019.00099.

Julier, A. 2019. "Critiquing Hegemony, Creating Food, Crafting Justice: Cultivating an Activist Feminist Food Studies." In *Feminist Food Studies*, edited by B. Parker, J. Brady, E. Power & S. Belyea. Women's Press.

Ka Hei. 2014. Hawai'i Department of Education. https://hawaiipublicschools.org/

Kahakalau, K. 2019. "Mā'awe Pono: A Hawaiian Research Methodology." In *The Past Before Us: Mo'okū'auhau as Metholodogy*, edited by N. Wilson-Hokowhitu. University of Hawai'i Press.

Kame'eleihiwa, L. 1999. *Nā Wāhine Kapu: Divine Hawaiian Women*. 'Ai Pōhaku Press.

Kauanui, J.K. 2008. *Hawaiian Blood: Colonialism and the Politics of Sovereignty and Indigeneity*. Duke University Press.

Kawelo, H. 2016. "Hi'ilei Kawelo Vignette." In *Food and Power in Hawai'i: Visions of Food Democracy*, edited by A.H. Kimura & K. Suryanata. University of Hawai'i Press.

Kenner, R., Pearlstein, E., Roberts, K., Schlosser, E., Pollan, M., Hirshberg, G. & Salatin, J. 2009. *Food, Inc.* [Motion Picture]. Magnolia Home Entertainment.

Kimmerer, R.W. 2013. *Braiding Sweetgrass: Indigenous Wisdom, Scientific Knowledge, and the Teachings of Plants.* Milkweed Editions.

Kimura, A.H. 2012. "Feminist Heuristics: Transforming the Foundation of Food Quality and Safety Assurance Systems." *Rural Sociology* 77 (2): 203–224. https://doi.org/10.1111/j.1549-0831.2012.00075.x.

Kirwan, J. 2004. "Alternative Strategies in the UK Agro-Food System: Interrogating the Alterity of Farmers' Markets." *Sociologia Ruralis* 44 (4): 395–415. https://doi.org/10.1111/j.1467-9523.2004.00283.x.

Kneen, C. 2011. "We Can Do It!" In Saul, N., Kneen, C., Cyr, C., Fraser, E., Rimas, A., Thompson, S., Gulrukh, A., Murthy, A., Beaton, S., Diamant, S., Ekoko, B. E., Atkinson, L., Rao, A., Desjardins, E., Scott, S., Lister, N.-M., & Alton, C. , contributors to Revolutionary Fodder. *Alternatives Journal* 37 (2): 12. http://www.jstor.org/stable/45033995.

Kodama-Nishimoto, M. ed. 1996. *Hanahana: An Oral History Anthology of Hawaiʻi's Working People.* University of Hawaiʻi Press.

Kōkua Hawaiʻi Foundation. 2022. "Mission statement." https://kokuahawaii-foundation.org/about-us/.

Kuahiwi Ranch. 2024. "Kuahiwi Ranch: About Us." https://kuahiwi.com/.

Kuhnlein, H. 2017. "Gender Roles, Food System Biodiversity, and Food Security in Indigenous Peoples' Communities." *Maternal & Child Nutrition* 13 (3): 1–5. https://doi.org/10.1111/mcn.12529.

Kunze, J. 2023. "In the Extinction Capital of the World, a Native School is Restoring Indigenous Forests." *Native News Online*, March 21. https://native-newsonline.net/environment/school-restoring-indigenous-forests.

Kuo, H.J. & Peters, D.J. 2017. "The Socioeconomic Geography of Organic Agriculture in the United States." *Agroecology and Sustainable Food Systems* 41 (9–10): 1162–1184. https://doi.org/10.1080/21683565.2017.1359808.

LaDuke, W. 1999. *All Our Relations: Native Struggles for Land and Life.* South End Press.

LaDuke, W. 2005. *Recovering the Sacred: The Power of Naming and Claiming.* South End Press.

LaDuke, W. 2012. "Seeds of Our Ancestors, Seeds of Life." *TEDx Talks.* https://www.youtube.com/watch?v=pHNlel72eQc.

LaJeunesse, S. 2018. Eruption. *University of Hawai'i Sea Grant.* https://seagrant.soest.hawaii.edu/eruption/.

Latest Treaty Settlement Bill. 2019. "Treaty Settlement Bills Open for Submissions." July 25. https://www.parliament.nz/mi/get-involved/features/latest-treaty-settlement-bill/.

Latif, J. 2020. "The Story Behind the Fight to Save Ihumātao." *The Spinoff.* https://thespinoff.co.nz/atea/18-12-2020/the-story-behind-the-fight-to-save-ihumatao.

La Via Campesina. 2007. "Declaration of Nyéléni." https://viacampesina.org/en/what-is-food-sovereignty/.

Lemke, S. & Delormier, T. 2017. "Indigenous Peoples' Food Systems, Nutrition, and Gender: Conceptual and Methodological Considerations." *Maternal & Child Nutrition* 13 (3): 1–12. https://doi.org/10.1111/mcn.12499.

Leone, D. 2006. "State High Court Upholds Study for Koa Ridge Plan." *Honolulu Star-Bulletin.* https://www.hawaii.edu/ohelo/recent_developments_articles/koa_ridge_EA_ruling.htm.

Leung, P. & Loke, M. 2008. *Economic Impacts of Increasing Hawai'i's Food Self-Sufficiency.* Cooperative Extension Service: College of Tropical Agriculture and Human Resources—University of Hawai'i at Mānoa.

Little, J., Ilbery, B. & Watts, D. 2009. "Gender, Consumption and the Relocalisation of Food: A Research Agenda." *Sociologia Ruralis* 49 (3): 201–217. https://doi.org/10.1111/j.1467-9523.2009.00492.x.

Lobao, L. & Meyer, K. 1995. "Economic Decline, Gender and Labor Flexibility in Family-Based Enterprises: Midwestern Farming in the 1980s." *Social Forces* 74 (2): 575-608. https://doi.org/10.2307/2580493.

Local Food Production Dashboard. 2025. "Local Food Production and Consumption." https://alohachallenge.hawaii.gov/pages/local-food-production-and-consumption.

Lorde, A. 1984. "The Master's Tools Will Never Dismantle the Master's House." In *Sister Outsider: Essays and Speeches.* Crossing Press.

Lundahl, A. 2017. "Shifting Food Consciousness: Homesteading Blogs and the Inner Work of Food." *International Review of Social Research* 7(2): 80-89. https://doi.org/10.1515/irsr-2017-0010.

Lyte, B. 2021. "How Hawaii Squandered its Food Security—And What It Will Take to Get it Back." *Honolulu Civil Beat*, April 23. https://www.civilbeat.org/2021/04/how-hawaii-squandered-its-food-security-and-what-it-will-take-to-get-it-back/.

Lyver, P.O'B., Timoti, P., Gormley, A. et al. 2017. "Key Māori Values Strengthen the Mapping of Forest Ecosystem Services." *Ecosystem Services* 27: 92–102. https://doi.org/10.1016/j.ecoser.2017.08.009.

Maui Nui Venison. 2025. "Mission Statement." https://mauinuivenison.com/pages/mission.

McGregor, L.W. 2018. "How Food Secure Are We If Natural Disaster Strikes?" University of Hawai'i Sea Grant. https://seagrant.soest.hawaii.edu/how-food-secure-are-we-if-natural-disaster-strikes/.

McIntyre, B., Herren, H., Wakhungu, J. & Watson, R. eds. 2009. *International Assessment of Agricultural Knowledge, Science and Technology for Development.* Island Press.

McKay, G. 2011. *Radical Gardening: Politics, Idealism & Rebellion in the Garden.* Frances Lincoln—Distributed by PGW.

Meares, A. C. 1997. "Making the Transition from Conventional to Sustainable Agriculture: Gender, Social Movement Participation, and Quality of Life on the Family Farm." *Rural Sociology* 62 (1): 21-47. https://doi.org/10.1111/j.1549-0831.1997.tb00643.x.

Melnychuk, M.C., Peterson, E., Elliott, M. & Hilborn, R. 2017. "Fisheries Management Impacts on Target Species Status." *Proceedings of the National Academy of Sciences* 114 (1) 178-183. https://doi.org/10.1073/pnas.1609915114.

Mello, C., King, L.O. & Adams, I. 2017. "Growing Food, Growing Consciousness: Gardening and Social Justice in Grand Rapids, Michigan." *Culture, Agriculture, Food and Environment* 39 (2): 143–147. https://doi.org/10.1111/cuag.12091.

Meyer, M. 2019. "'Aha 'Imi Na'auao: Hawaiian Knowing and Wellbeing: Research and Community Collaboration to Affirm the Qualities of Hawaiian Health and Wellness." https://westoahu.hawaii.edu/ekamakanihou/?p=9855.

Mikaere, A. 2019. "Colonisation and the Imposition of Patriarchy: A Ngāti Raukawa Woman's Perspective." In *Mana Wahine Reader: A Collection of Writings 1999–2019*, vol. II, edited by L. Pihama, L. Tuhiwai Smith, N. Simmonds, J. Seed-Pihama & K. Gabel. Te Kotahi Research Institute.

Ministry for Primary Industries. 2025. "Māori Customary Fishing Information and Resources." *Fisheries New Zealand*. https://www.mpi.govt.nz/fishing-aquaculture/ maori-customary-fishing/maori-customary-fishing-information-and-resources/.

Mironesco, M. 2016. Farmers' Markets in Hawai'i. In *Food and Power in Hawai'i: Visions of Food Democracy,* edited by A.H. Kimura & K. Suryanata. University of Hawai'i Press.

Mischan, L. 2022. "How to Turn the Humble Lentil into an Extravagant Luxury." *New York Times*. https://www.nytimes.com/2022/03/23/magazine/lentil-stew.html.

Mitra, I. 2021. "Analysing bell hook's Essay on Marginality from Sandra Harding's *Feminist Standpoint Theory Reader*." *Feminism in India.* https://feminisminindia. com/2021/11/16/bell-hooks-margin-sandra-harding-feminist-standpoint-theory/.

Mo Hiakai. 2022. "About: Hiakai NZ." https://www.hiakai.co.nz/about.

Moeke-Pickering, T., Heitia, M., Heitia, S., Karapu, R. & Cote-Meek, S. 2015. "Understanding Māori Food Security and Food Sovereignty Issues in Whakatāne." *MAI Journal* 4 (1): 29–42. https://www.journal.mai.ac.nz/content/ understanding-māori-food-security-and-food-sovereignty-issues-whakatāne.

Mohanty, C. 1984. "Under Western Eyes: Feminist Scholarship and Colonial Discourses." *Feminist Review* 30: 61-88. https://doi.org/10.1057/fr.1988.42.

Mollett, S. & Faria, C. 2013. "Messing with Gender in Feminist Political Ecology." *Geoforum* 45: 116–125. https://doi.org/10.1016/j.geoforum.2012.10.009.

Moorfield, J.C. 2024. *Te Aka Māori-English, English-Māori Dictionary and Index*. https://maoridictionary.co.nz

Moreton-Robinson, A. 2015. *The White Possessive: Property, Power, and Indigenous Sovereignty.* University of Minnesota Press.

Morrison, D. 2011. "Indigenous Food Sovereignty: A Model for Social Learning." In *Food Sovereignty in Canada: Creating Just and Sustainable Food Systems*, edited by H. Wittman, A. Desmarais, & N. Wiebe. Fernwood.

Moss, R.L. 2025. "Healthy Children Become Healthy Adults." *Nemours Children's Health.* https://www.nemours.org/well-beyond-medicine/leadership-in-redefining-childrens-health/healthy-children-become-healthy-adults.html.

Mpfou, E. 2020. "Keeping the Struggles of Peasant Women Alive." *La Via Campesina*, August 6. https://viacampesina.org/en/keeping-the-struggles-of-peasant-women-alive-2/ .

Mulaney, E. G. 2014. "Geopolitical Maize: Peasant Seeds, Everyday Practices, and Food Security in Mexico." *Geopolitics* 19: 406–430. https://doi.org/10.10 80/14650045.2014.920232.

Naranjo, A., Johnson, A., Rossow, H. & Kebreab, E. 2020. "Greenhouse Gas, Water, and Land Footprint per Unit of Production of the California Dairy Industry over 50 years." *Journal of Dairy Science* 103 (4): 3760-3773. https://doi.org/10.3168/jds.2019-16576.

National Institute of Food and Agriculture. 2025. "Importance of Sustainable Agriculture." https://www.nifa.usda.gov/topics/sustainable-agriculture.

National Tropical Botanical Garden. 2020. "About Breadfruit." https://ntbg .org/breadfruit/about-breadfruit/.

Natural Resources Defense Council. 2020. "Industrial Agriculture 101." https://www.nrdc.org/stories/industrial-agriculture-101.

Natural Resources Defense Council. 2021. "What is Regenerative Agriculture?" https://www.nrdc.org/stories/regenerative-agriculture-101.

Neff, R., Palmer, A., McKenzie, S. & Lawrence, R. 2009. "Food Systems and Public Health Disparities." *Journal of Hunger and Environmental Nutrition* 4: 282–314. https://doi.org/10.1080/19320240903337041.

New Zealand Productivity Commission. 2020. "The Dairy Sector in New Zealand: Extending the Boundaries." https://www.tdb.co.nz/dairy-sector-extending-the-boundaries/.

Ng, R. 2022. "Hawaiian Foodways are Vanishing: Chef Brian Hirata Won't Let That Happen." *Bon Appétit*, May 19. https://www.bonappetit.com/hawaii-chef-brian-hirata-foraging-native-ingredients.

Nigh, R. & Gonzáles Cabañas, A.A. 2015. "Reflexive Consumer Markets as Opportunities for New Peasant Farmers in Mexico and France: Constructing Food

Sovereignty through Alternative Food Networks." *Agroecology and Sustainable Food Systems* 39: 317–341. https://doi.org/10.1080/21683565.2014.973545.

Norgaard, K.M. 2019. *Salmon and Acorns Feed Our People: Colonialism, Nature & Social Action.* Rutgers University Press.

Nosowitz, D. 2021. "The Struggle to Contain, and Eat, the Invasive Deer Taking over Hawaiʻi." *Modern Farmer*, May 24. https://modernfarmer.com/2021/05/the-struggle-to-contain-and-eat-the-invasive-deer-taking-over-hawaii/.

Office of Hawaiian Affairs. 2024. "Island Community Report: Molokaʻi." Office of Research and Evaluation. https://www.oha.org/wp-content/uploads/2024-Molo-kai-Island-Community-Report.pdf.

Okamura, J. 2024. "Hawaii Should Stop Pretending It's a Multicultural Paradise." *Honolulu Civil Beat.* https://www.civilbeat.org/2024/06/jonathan-okamura-hawaii-should-stop-pretending-its-a-multicultural-paradise/.

Oliver, B. 2016. "'The Earth Gives Us So Much': Agroecology and Rural Women's Leadership in Uruguay." *Culture, Agriculture, Food and Environment* 38 (1): 38–47. https://doi.org/10.1111/cuag.12064.

Olsen, B. 2020. "NZ Continues to Produce and Import Food, So There's No Need to Panic Buy." *Infometrics New Zealand.* https://www.infometrics.co.nz/article/2020-03-nz-continues-to-produce-and-import-food-so-theres-no-need-to-panic-buy.

Ostrander, M. 2011. "Joel Salatin: How to Eat Animals and Respect Them, Too." *Yes Magazine*, March 28. https://www.yesmagazine.org/issue/animals/2011/03/28/joel-salatin-how-to-eat-meat-and-respect-it-too.

Park, C.M.Y., White, B., & Julia. 2015. "We Are Not All the Same: Taking Gender Seriously in Food Sovereignty Discourse." *Third World Quarterly* 36 (3): 584–599. https://doi.org/10.1080/01436597.2015.1002988.

Patel, R.C. 2012. "Food Sovereignty: Power, Gender, and the Right to Food." *PLoS Medicine* 9 (6): 1-4. https://doi.org/10.1371/journal.pmed.1001223.

Paulin, C.D. 2007. "Perspectives on Māori Fishing History and Technique. Ngā āhua me ngā pūrākau me ngā hangarau ika o te Māori. *Tuhinga* 18: 11-47. https://natlib-primo.hosted.exlibrisgroup.com/permalink/f/1fro764/INNZ7118295720002837.

Pereira, P.M. & Vicente, A.F. 2013. "Meat Nutritional Composition and Nutritive Role in the Human Diet." *Meat Science* 93 (3): 586–592. https://doi .org/10.1016/j.meatsci.2012.09.018.

Peterson, C. & Mitloehner, F. 2021. "Sustainability of the Dairy Industry: Emissions and Mitigation Opportunities." *Frontiers in Animal Science* 2: 1–11. https://doi.org/10.3389/fanim.2021.760310.

Pihama, L. 2019. "Mana Wahine Theory: Creating Space for Māori Women's Theories." In *Mana Wahine Reader: A Collection of Writings 1999–2019*, vol. II, edited by Pihama, L., Tuhiwai Smith, L., Simmonds, N., Seed-Pihama, J. & Gabel, K. eds. Te Kotahi Research Institute.

Pihama, L., Tuhiwai Smith, L., Simmonds, N., Seed-Pihama, J. & Gabel, K. eds 2019a. *Mana Wahine Reader: A Collection of Writings 1987–1998*, vol. I. Te Kotahi Research Institute.

Pihama, L., Tuhiwai Smith, L., Simmonds, N., Seed-Pihama, J. & Gabel, K. eds. 2019b. *Mana Wahine Reader: A Collection of Writings 1999–2019*, vol. II. Te Kotahi Research Institute.

Pimbert, M. 2009. "Women and Food Sovereignty." *LEISA Magazine* 25 (3): 6–9. https://www.yumpu.com/en/document/view/34619823/women-and-food-sovereignty-leisa-india.

Pollan, M. 2006. *Omnivore's Dilemma: A Natural History of Four Meals*. Penguin.

Pukui, M.K. 1983. *'Ōlelo No'eau: Hawaiian Proverbs & Poetical Sayings*. Bishop Museum Press.

Red Nation. 2021. *The Red Deal: Indigenous Action to Save Our Earth*. Common Notions.

Rich, A. 1978. *The Dream of a Common Language: Poems 1974–1977*. WW Norton.

Rich, A. 1986. "Notes Towards a Politics of Location." In *Blood, Bread, and Poetry: Selected Prose 1979–1985*. Norton.

Ripeka-Evans. 2019. "The Negation of Powerlessness: Māori Feminism, a Perspective." In *Mana Wahine Reader: A Collection of Writings 1987–1998*, vol. I, edited by L. Pihama, L. Tuhiwai Smith, N. Simmonds, J. Seed-Pihama & K. Gabel. Te Kotahi Research Institute.

Robinson, M. 2013. "Veganism and Mi'kmaq Legends." *Canadian Journal of Native Studies* 33 (1): 189-196. https://doi.org/10.4324/9781003013891-4.

Rochelau, D. & Nirmal, P. 2014. "Feminist Political Ecologies: Grounded, Networked and Rooted on Earth." In *The Oxford Handbook on Transnational Feminism*, edited by R. Baksh & W. Harcourt. Oxford University Press.

Rochelau, D., Thomas-Slayter, B. & Wangari, E. 1996. *Feminist Political Ecology: Global Issues and Local Experience*. Routledge.

Roskruge, N. 2009. "Tāhuri Whenua Bringing Māori Growers Together." *Science Learning Hub: Pokapū Akoranga Pūtaio*. https://www.sciencelearn.org.nz/videos/387-tahuri-whenua-bringing-maori-growers-together.

Rudolph, K.R., & McLachlan, S.M. 2013. "Seeking Indigenous Food Sovereignty: Origins of and Responses to the Food Crisis in Northern Manitoba, Canada." *Local Environment* 18 (9): 1079–1098. https://doi.org/10.1080/13549839.2012.754741.

Rudy, K. 2011. *Loving Animals: Toward a New Animal Advocacy*. University of Minnesota Press.

Sachs, C. E. 1996. *Gendered Fields: Rural Women, Agriculture, and Environment*. Westview Press.

Sachs, C. & Patel-Campillo, A. 2014. "Feminist Food Justice: Crafting a New Vision." *Feminist Studies* 40 (2): 396-410. https://doi.org/10.1353/fem.2014.0008.

San Diego Foundation. 2022. "What Is Food Sovereignty?" https://www.sdfoundation.org/news-events/sdf-news/what-is-food-sovereignty/.

de Schutter, O. 2013. "The Agrarian Transition and the "Feminization" of Agriculture." In *Food Sovereignty: A Critical Dialogue*. https://www.tni.org/en/publication/the-agrarian-transition-and-the-feminization-of-agriculture.

Serrato, C. 2021. "Reality Bites with Claudia Serrato." *Passerby Magazine*. https://passerbymagazine.com/profiles/claudia-serrato.

Shapiro, T. 2013. "Hurdles Cleared for Ho'opili, Koa Ridge." *Honolulu Magazine*. https://www.honolulumagazine.com/hurdles-cleared-for-hoopili-koa-ridge/.

Shattuck, A., Schiavoni, C.M., & Van Gelder, Z. 2015. "Translating the Politics of Food Sovereignty: Digging into Contradictions, Uncovering New Dimensions." *Globalizations* 12 (4): 421–433. https://doi.org/10.1080/14747731.2015.1041243.

Sherman, S. 2022. "One Sioux Chef's Attempt to Reclaim Native American Cuisine." TED Radio Hour Comics. https://www.npr.org/2022/05/13/1097955036/comic-one-sioux-chefs-attempt-to-reclaim-native-american-cuisine.

Shirley, L. 2013. "Is Māori Food Sovereignty Affected by Adherence, or Lack Thereof, to Te Tiriti O Waitangi?" *Future of Food: Journal on Food, Agriculture, and Society* 1 (2): 57–63. ISSN-Internet: 2197-411X / OCLC-Nr.: 862804632

Shiva, V. 1988. *Staying Alive.* Zed Books.

Shiva, V., and M. Mies. 1993. *Ecofeminism.* Zed Books.

Shoemaker, N. 2015. "A Typology of Colonialism." *Perspectives on History*, October 1. https://www.historians.org/research-and-publications/perspectives-on-history/october-2015/a-typology-of-colonialism.

Silva, N. 2004. *Aloha Betrayed: Native Hawaiian Resistance to American Colonialism.* Duke University Press.

Simpson, L. 2017. *As We Have Always Done: Indigenous Freedom and Radical Resistance.* University of Minnesota Press.

Slocum, R. 2007. "Whiteness, Space and Alternative Food Practice." *Geoforum* 38 (3): 520–533. https://doi.org/10.1016/j.geoforum.2006.10.006.

Slooten, E., Simmons, G., Dawson, S.M., Bremner, G, Thrush, S.F., Whittaker, H., McCormack, F., Robertson, B.C., Haworth, N., Clarke, P.J., Pauly, D. & Zeller, D. 2017. "Evidence of Bias in Assessment of Fisheries Management Impacts." *Proceedings of the National Academy of Sciences.* 114 (25) E4901-E4902, https://doi.org/10.1073/pnas.1706544114.

Smith, L.T. 1999. *Decolonizing Methodologies: Research and Indigenous Peoples,* 1st edition. Zed Books.

Spivak, G. 1985. "Criticism, Feminism and the Institution: An Interview with Gayatri Chakravorty Spivak." *Thesis Eleven*, vol. 10-11 (1): 175–87. https://doi.org/10.1177/072551368501000113.

Stein, K., Mirosa, M. & Carter, L. 2018. "Māori Women Leading Local Sustainable Food Systems." *AlterNative* 14 (2): 147–155. https://doi.org/10.1177/1177180117753168.

Steiner, R. 1993. *Agriculture: Spiritual Foundations for Renewal of Agriculture.* Biodynamic Association.

Stevenson, S. 2011. *Edible Impact: Food Security Policy Literature Review.* Toi Te Ora—Public Health Service, BOPDHB.

Storhaug, C.L., Fosse, S.K. & Fadnes, L.T. 2017. "Country, Regional, and Global Estimates for Lactose Malabsorption in Adults: A Systematic Review and Meta-Analysis." *Lancet: Gastroenterology & Hepatology* 2 (10): 738–746. https://doi.org/10.1016/S2468-1253(17)30154-1.

Sundberg, J. 2017. "Feminist Political Ecology." In *International Encyclopedia of Geography: People, the Earth, Environment and Technology*, edited by D. Richardson, N. Castree, M. Goodchild, A. Kobayashi, W. Liu, & R. Marston. Wiley-Blackwell.

Slaughter, A-M. 2015. *Unfinished Business: Women, Men, Work, Family.* Random House.

Szalai, J. 2015. "The Complicated Origins of "'Having It All.'" *New York Times.* https://www.nytimes.com/2015/01/04/magazine/the-complicated-origins-of-having-it-all.html

Taonui, R. 2020. "The Argument for Māori Women Speaking on the Marae." *The Spinoff.* https://thespinoff.co.nz/atea/13-03-2020/the-argument-for-maori-women-speaking-on-the-marae.

Tavenner, K., Crane, T.A., Bullock, R., & Galiè, A. 2022. "Intersectionality in Gender and Agriculture: Toward an Applied Research Design." *Gender, Technology and Development* 26 (3): 385–403. https://doi.org/10.1080/09718 524.2022.2140383.

Te Ahukaramū, C.R. 2007a. "Kaitiakitanga—Guardianship and Conservation— Kaitiakitanga Today." *Te Ara—The Encyclopedia of New Zealand.* https://teara. govt.nz/en/kaitiakitanga-guardianship-and-conservation/page-7.

Te Ahukaramū, C. R. 2007b. "Papatūānuku—the Land." *Te Ara—The Encyclopedia of New Zealand.* https://teara.govt.nz/en/papatuanuku-the-land.

Te Awekotuku, N. 1991. "He Whiriwhiri Wahine: Framing Women's Studies for Aotearoa." In *Mana Wahine Reader: A Collection of Writings 1987–1998*, vol. I, edited by L. Pihama, L. Tuhiwai Smith, N. Simmonds, J. Seed-Pihama & K. Gabel. Te Kotahi Research Institute.

Te Morenga, L. 2017. *A Kaupapa Māori co-design approach for developing a healthy lifestyle support tool for use in New Zealand Māori communities.* University of Otago.

Te Ohu Kaimoana. 2017. "Post Election Briefing." *Te Ohu Kaimoana.* https://www.teohukaimoana.nz/reports/te-ohu-kaimoana-briefing-to-the-incoming-minister-for-oceans-and-fisheries-2017.

Te Tai—Treaty Settlement Stories. 2020. "What Are Treaty Settlements and Why Are They Needed?" https://teara.govt.nz/en/te-tai/about-treaty-settlements.

Tengan, T. K. 2008. *Native Men Remade: Gender and Nation in Contemporary Hawai'i.* Duke University Press.

Tennant, M., O'Brien, M. & Sanders, J. 2008. *The History of the Non-Profit Sector in New Zealand.* Office for the Community & Voluntary Sector: Tari mō te Rāngai ā-Hapori, ā-Tūao.

Terrell, J. 2021. "Hawaii's Food System is Broken: Now Is the Time to Fix It." *Honolulu Civil Beat.* https://www.civilbeat.org/2021/01/hawaiis-food-system-is-broken-now-is-the-time-to-fix-it/.

Thirkill, M. 2021. "Racism on the Scales." *Public Health Post.* https://publichealthpost.org/health-equity/racism-bmi/.

Trask, H.K. 1991. "Lovely Hula Hands: Corporate Tourism and the Prostitution of Hawaiian Culture." *Contours* 5 (1): 8–14. https://www.cabidigitallibrary.org/doi/full/10.5555/19911887773.

Trask, H.K. 1993. *From a Native Daughter: Colonialism and Sovereignty in Hawai'i.* University of Hawai'i Press.

Trauger, A. 2004. "'Because They Can Do the Work': Women Farmers in Sustainable Agriculture in Pennsylvania." *Gender, Place and Culture* 11 (2): 290–307. https://doi.org/10.1080/0966369042000218491.

Tuhiwai Smith, L. 2019. "Getting Out from Down Under: Māori Women, Education, and the Struggles for Mana Wahine." In *Mana Wahine Reader: A Collection of Writings 1987–1998*, vol. I, edited by L. Pihama, L. Tuhiwai Smith, N. Simmonds, J. Seed-Pihama & K. Gabel. Te Kotahi Research Institute.

United Nations Food and Agriculture Organization. 2013. "Tackling Climate Change through Livestock: A Global Assessment of Emissions and Mitigation Opportunities." https://www.fao.org/4/i3437e/i3437e00.htm.

US Census 2022 Community Resilience Estimates. 2022. "US Climate Resilience Toolkit." https://toolkit.climate.gov/tool/us-census-2022-community-resilience-estimates

Vandevijvere, S., Mackay, S., D'Souza, E. & Swinburn, B. 2019. "The First INFORMAS National Food Environments and Policies Survey in New Zealand: A Blueprint Country Profile for Measuring Progress on Creating Healthy Food Environments." *Obesity Reviews* 20 (S2): 141–160. https://doi.org/10.1111/obr.12850.

Venn, L., Kneafsey, M., Cox, L.H.R., Dowler, E. & Tuomainen, H. 2006. "Researching European 'Alternative' Food Networks: Some Methodological Considerations." *Area* 38: 248–348. https://doi.org/10.1111/j.1475-4762.2006.00694.x.

Veracini, L. 2010. *Settler Colonialism: A Theoretical Overview.* Springer

Voth, K. & Gilker, R. 2017. "What 30 Years of Study Tell us about Grazing and Carbon Sequestration." *On Pasture.* https://onpasture.com/2017/11/13/what-30-years-of-study-tell-us-about-grazing-and-carbon-sequestration/.

Wahl, D., Villinger, K., König, L.M., Ziesemer, K., Schupp, H.T. & Renner, B. 2017. "Healthy Food Choices Are Happy Food Choices: Evidence from a Real-Life Sample Using Smartphone-Based Assessments." *Scientific Reports* 7 (1): 17069. https://doi.org/10.1038/s41598-017-17262-9.

Waitere, H. & Johnson, P. 2019. "Echoed Silences in Absentia: Mana Wahine in Institutional Contexts." In *Mana Wahine Reader: A Collection of Writings 1999–2019*, vol. II, edited by L. Pihama, L. Tuhiwai Smith, N. Simmonds, J. Seed-Pihama, & K. Gabel. Te Kotahi Research Institute.

Weigert, P. 2025. "Feeding Hawai'i: Portraits of Resilience." https://feeding-hawaii.squarespace.com/talkstory/pomai-weigert.

Westervelt, E. 2020. "During Pandemic, Community Supported Agriculture Sees Membership Spike." *National Public Radio.* https://www.npr.org/2020/05/14/855855756/as-pandemic-devastates-economy-community-supported-agriculture-sees-membership-s.

Whatmore, S. 1991. *Farming Women: Gender, Work, and Family Enterprise.* MacMillan.

Wiebe, N. & Wipf, K. 2011. "Nurturing Food Sovereignty in Canada." In *Food Sovereignty in Canada: Creating Just and Sustainable Food Systems*, edited by H. Wittman, A. Desmarais & N. Wiebe. Fernwood.

Wittman, H., Desmarais, A. & Wiebe, N. 2010. "The Origins and Potential of Food Sovereignty." In *Food Sovereignty: Reconnecting Food, Nature, and Community,* edited by H. Wittman, A. Desmarais & N. Wiebe. Fernwood Publishing.

World Health Organization. 2023. "WHO Updates Guidelines on Fats and Carbohydrates." *Health Topics.* https://www.who.int/news/item/17-07-2023-who-updates-guidelines-on-fats-and-carbohydrates.

Wyss, T'uy't'tana-Cease. 2019. Quoted in Duvauchelle, J. "Seeing Ethical Meat through an Indigenous Lens: Hunting for a More Sustainable Future." *Alive Magazine.* https://www.alive.com/lifestyle/seeing-ethical-meat-through-an-indigenous-lens/.

Yamashiro, A. & N. Goodyear-Kaʻōpua, eds. 2014. *The Value of Hawaiʻi: Ancestral Roots, Oceanic Visions*, vol. 2. University of Hawaiʻi Press.

Yamashita, S.H. 2019. *Hawaiʻi Regional Cuisine: The Food Movement that Changed the Way Hawaiʻi Eats.* University of Hawaiʻi Press.

Younging, G. 2018. *Elements of Indigenous Style: A Guide for Writing by and About Indigenous Peoples*. Brush Education.

INDEX

matrix of domination, 14–15
meat, fish, and dairy, producing and
        consuming, 151–156. *See also*
        local meat, fish, and dairy
    alternative food movements, 160
    dairy, 165–167
    intersectional politics of, 157–165
    Kanaka Maoli diet, 159
    weighing the values of, 151–169
"Mother Earth" metaphor, 12

N
Native Hawaiian genealogy, 10
Native sovereignty, ix
networks of knowledge, 113–115
    humanizing systems, need for, 115
    nutrition and environment connection,
        122–124

O
Oddom, Ka'iulani, 35
Oi Collective women group, 31
'Ōlelo Hawai'i (Hawaiian language), vii
"our sea of islands" phenomenon, 35

P
Pākehā, political actors, 104
PermaDynamics, 66, 127
plant-based diets, weighing the values of,
        151–169
    agribusiness, 160
    veganism as a practice, 158
policy change creation through gifting,
        175–182
    allyship and activism, 177
    anti-GMO cause, 178
    female activists in, 178–179
    garden education curriculum, 180
    iwi tribes in, 182
    nonprofit organizations in, 181–182
    Polynesian-style, 179
    traditional ecological knowledge
        importance, 180–181

political engagement and food
        sovereignty, 7–9
political imagination, 26
Polynesian Triangle, 36
positionality and practice, 20–25
protein consumption, nutrition, and
        public health, 167–169

R
Red New Deal, 27

S
school food movement, 99
School Garden Hui network, 95
school lunch, 117–122
    cafeteria scratch cooking, 118
    decolonizing diets, 122
    during COVID-19 pandemic, 121
    growing own food, 120
settler colonialism, xiii
sharing abundance with others, 173
Silva, N., viii
Slow Food movement, 22
social norming, 179
Spira NZ, 101
stories as seeds of change, 187–194
    food system as a space of resistance, 189
    gendered attitudes toward work, 190
    idea of home and mothering
        conception, 193
    potential for exchange, 188
    systems-thinking, 186–187, 190
success, redefining, 194–198
Supplemental Nutrition Assistance
        Program (SNAP), 70, 144
sustainable agriculture, 74–79
    food and family relationship
        importance in, 83–84
    importance of policy in, 75
    land and people relationship
        importance in, 77–78
    scientific basis of Native agricultural
        practices, 76

www.ingramcontent.com/pod-product-compliance
Lightning Source LLC
Chambersburg PA
CBHW031550260326
41914CB00002B/356